IBS DIET

COOKBOOK

Discover the Low-FODMAP Plan for a life-changing benefit of Gut-Friendly Recipes to Ease the Symptoms of IBS, and Other Digestive Disorders

MONALISA BLAKE

Table of Contents

INTRODUCTION

Irritable bowel syndrome (IBS) is a condition affecting the gastrointestinal system and is one of the most common conditions to affect the digestive system. It is a long-term condition and is characterized by abdominal pain, bloating, and altered bowel habits. It is a disorder that is not life-threatening and does not lead to a serious disease such as cancer. It is, however, a chronic condition that can cause considerable discomfort and distress. People with IBS commonly feel they have to "live" with their condition. This can have an impact on their quality of life as IBS can affect social, work, and domestic activities. Irritable Bowel Syndrome (IBS) has long been a challenging condition to manage effectively, characterized by a complex interplay of symptoms including abdominal pain, bloating, and altered bowel habits. However, recent years have witnessed a remarkable revolution in the treatment landscape of IBS, marked by innovative therapies, enhanced understanding of the condition, and a patient-centric approach. This article delves into the advancements in IBS treatment, their efficacy, and the promising future prospects they hold.

Advancements in Pharmacotherapy: Traditional pharmacological interventions for IBS primarily targeted symptom relief, often with limited success and significant side effects. However, the advent of novel pharmacotherapeutic agents has transformed the treatment paradigm. One notable development is the introduction of gut-targeted therapies, such as rifaximin, which selectively modulates gut microbiota and has shown efficacy in alleviating IBS symptoms, particularly diarrhea-predominant IBS (IBS-D). Additionally, drugs targeting visceral hypersensitivity, serotonin receptors, and motility regulators have expanded the therapeutic armamentarium, offering tailored approaches for different subtypes of IBS.

Biopsychosocial Approaches: Recognizing the multifactorial nature of IBS, there has been a paradigm shift towards biopsychosocial models of care. Cognitive-behavioral therapy (CBT), hypnotherapy, and mindfulness-based interventions have emerged as effective adjuncts to pharmacotherapy, addressing the psychological and emotional components of IBS while fostering self-management skills and resilience. Moreover, the integration of dietary modifications, probiotics, and lifestyle interventions underscores the holistic approach to managing IBS, empowering patients to actively participate in their treatment journey.

Precision Medicine and Personalized Therapies: The era of precision medicine has ushered in a new era of tailored therapies for IBS, leveraging advancements in genetics, microbiome profiling, and biomarker discovery. Through genetic testing and microbiome analysis, clinicians can identify individualized risk factors and treatment responses, paving the way for personalized pharmacotherapy and dietary interventions. Furthermore, the advent of fecal microbiota transplantation (FMT) holds promise in restoring gut dysbiosis and alleviating IBS symptoms, although further research is warranted to elucidate its long-term efficacy and safety profile.

Patient-Centric Care and Shared Decision-Making: Central to the revolution in IBS treatment is a paradigm shift towards patient-centric care and shared decision-making. Empowering patients with education, support, and self-management strategies fosters a collaborative approach to treatment, enhancing treatment adherence and patient satisfaction. Moreover, patient advocacy groups and online communities play a pivotal role in raising awareness, reducing stigma, and advocating for research funding and policy changes to improve IBS care globally.

Future Directions and Challenges: Looking ahead, the future of IBS treatment holds immense promise, fueled by ongoing research into novel therapeutic targets, biomarkers, and non-invasive diagnostic tools. Advances in neurogastroenterology, artificial intelligence, and digital health technologies offer exciting opportunities for personalized, precision-based interventions tailored to the unique needs of each patient. However, challenges such as treatment access, healthcare disparities, and the need for interdisciplinary collaboration underscore the importance of continued advocacy, research, and innovation in the field of gastroenterology.

The revolution in IBS treatment heralds a new era of hope and optimism for millions of individuals worldwide grappling with this debilitating condition. From pharmacological innovations to biopsychosocial interventions and personalized therapies, the evolving treatment landscape underscores the importance of a multidimensional approach to IBS care. By embracing patient-centric principles, advancing scientific knowledge, and fostering collaboration across disciplines, we can strive towards improving outcomes and quality of life for individuals living with IBS.

UNDERSTANDING IBS

IBS is a complex gastrointestinal disorder characterized by a diverse array of symptoms, including abdominal pain, bloating, altered bowel habits, and discomfort. These symptoms often fluctuate in severity and duration, significantly impacting the quality of life of affected individuals. While the exact etiology of IBS remains incompletely understood, it is believed to arise from a combination of genetic predisposition, environmental factors, gut dysmotility, visceral hypersensitivity, alterations in gut microbiota, and psychosocial influences.

Symptoms of IBS: The symptoms of IBS can vary widely among individuals and may include:

- Abdominal pain or discomfort, typically relieved by bowel movements

- Changes in bowel habits, such as diarrhea, constipation, or a mix of both

- Bloating and abdominal distension

- Excessive gas (flatulence)

- Mucus in the stool

These symptoms can profoundly impact daily life, leading to absenteeism from work or school, social withdrawal, and emotional distress. It is essential to recognize that the presentation of IBS can differ among populations and may be influenced by cultural, dietary, and lifestyle factors.

Diagnostic Approaches: Diagnosing IBS requires a thorough clinical evaluation, including a detailed medical history, physical examination, and exclusion of other organic gastrointestinal disorders. Key diagnostic criteria, such as the Rome criteria, aid in categorizing IBS based on symptom patterns and duration. Diagnostic tests may include:

- Laboratory investigations, including blood tests and stool studies, to rule out other conditions

- Imaging studies, such as colonoscopy or abdominal ultrasound, in select cases

- Hydrogen breath tests to assess for carbohydrate malabsorption and small intestinal bacterial overgrowth

- Symptom assessment using validated questionnaires to quantify symptom severity and impact on quality of life

It is imperative to approach the diagnosis of IBS with sensitivity and empathy, recognizing the potential psychosocial impact of the condition on patients.

Management Strategies: Management of IBS is multifaceted and tailored to individual patient needs, focusing on symptom relief, improvement of quality of life, and long-term management. Treatment strategies may include:

- Dietary modifications: Elimination or reduction of trigger foods, such as high-FODMAP foods, gluten, dairy, and spicy foods. The low-FODMAP diet, in particular, has shown efficacy in reducing IBS symptoms in some individuals.

- Pharmacotherapy: Symptom-specific medications, including antispasmodics, laxatives, anti-diarrheal agents, and antidepressants, may be prescribed based on predominant symptoms and patient response.

- Psychological interventions: Cognitive-behavioral therapy (CBT), gut-directed hypnotherapy, and relaxation techniques can help address the psychological aspects of IBS, such as anxiety, stress, and coping mechanisms.

- Lifestyle modifications: Regular exercise, adequate sleep, stress management techniques, and mindfulness practices can contribute to symptom improvement and overall well-being.

- Patient education and support: Providing patients with information about IBS, self-management strategies, and support resources, including patient advocacy groups and online communities, can empower individuals to actively participate in their care.

In refractory cases or when symptoms significantly impair quality of life, referral to a gastroenterologist or specialized IBS clinic may be warranted for further evaluation and consideration of advanced therapies, such as biofeedback, fecal microbiota transplantation (FMT), or investigational treatments.

Global Perspectives: IBS is a global health concern that transcends geographical boundaries, affecting individuals of all ages, genders, and ethnicities. While the prevalence and clinical presentation of IBS may vary among regions, the impact on patients' lives and the challenges in diagnosis and management remain universal. Cultural factors, dietary habits, healthcare access, and socioeconomic disparities can influence the experience of IBS and the availability of resources for its management.

In the USA, Europe, and other developed regions, efforts to raise awareness, improve access to care, and advance research into IBS are ongoing. Multidisciplinary approaches to IBS management, collaboration between healthcare providers and patient advocacy groups, and the integration of digital health technologies hold promise for enhancing patient outcomes and reducing the burden of IBS on healthcare systems.

CHAPTER ONE:

Diagnosis and Classification

Diagnosing and classifying Irritable Bowel Syndrome (IBS) is a multifaceted process that requires careful consideration of clinical symptoms, exclusion of other gastrointestinal disorders, and adherence to established diagnostic criteria. In this comprehensive overview, we will explore the various aspects of diagnosing and classifying IBS, including key diagnostic criteria, differential diagnosis, diagnostic tests, and subtyping of IBS based on symptom patterns.

Diagnostic Criteria: The diagnosis of IBS relies on established criteria that help differentiate it from other gastrointestinal disorders. The Rome criteria, developed by international expert consensus, are widely used for diagnosing functional gastrointestinal disorders, including IBS. The Rome IV criteria, the latest iteration, categorize IBS based on the presence of recurrent abdominal pain or discomfort at least once per week for the past three months, associated with two or more of the following:

1. Improvement with defecation

2. Onset associated with a change in frequency of stool

3. Onset associated with a change in form (appearance) of stool

These criteria help standardize the diagnosis of IBS and ensure consistency in clinical practice and research studies.

Differential Diagnosis:

One of the challenges in diagnosing IBS is differentiating it from other gastrointestinal disorders with similar symptoms. Conditions that may mimic IBS include:

1. Inflammatory Bowel Disease (IBD): Crohn's disease and ulcerative colitis can present with abdominal pain, diarrhea, and rectal bleeding, necessitating careful evaluation with endoscopic and histologic findings.

2. Celiac Disease: This autoimmune disorder characterized by gluten intolerance can manifest with diarrhea, abdominal pain, bloating, and malabsorption, requiring serologic testing and small intestinal biopsy for diagnosis.

3. Small Intestinal Bacterial Overgrowth (SIBO): Overgrowth of bacteria in the small intestine can lead to IBS-like symptoms, such as bloating, diarrhea, and malabsorption, necessitating breath testing for hydrogen or methane gas.

4. Colon Cancer: While less common, colon cancer can present with abdominal pain, changes in bowel habits, and rectal bleeding, warranting prompt evaluation with colonoscopy.

Diagnostic Tests:

Diagnostic testing in IBS is primarily aimed at excluding other gastrointestinal disorders and identifying potential contributing factors. Key diagnostic tests may include:

1. Laboratory Investigations: Blood tests to assess for inflammation (e.g., C-reactive protein, erythrocyte sedimentation rate) and screen for celiac disease (e.g., tissue transglutaminase antibodies).

2. Stool Studies: Analysis of stool samples for infectious pathogens (e.g., bacteria, parasites), fecal occult blood, and fecal calprotectin to evaluate for inflammation.

3. Imaging Studies: While not routinely indicated in all cases of IBS, imaging modalities such as colonoscopy, abdominal ultrasound, and computed tomography (CT) scans may be performed to evaluate for structural abnormalities or other gastrointestinal conditions.

It is important to individualize diagnostic testing based on clinical presentation, patient risk factors, and symptom severity, while minimizing unnecessary invasive procedures.

Subtyping of IBS:

IBS can be further classified into subtypes based on predominant bowel habits and stool consistency, which can guide treatment decisions and prognostication. The Manning criteria and the Bristol Stool Form Scale are commonly used to categorize IBS subtypes as follows:

1. IBS with Constipation (IBS-C): Predominant symptoms include constipation, straining during bowel movements, and hard or lumpy stools.

2. IBS with Diarrhea (IBS-D): Predominant symptoms include diarrhea, urgency, and loose or watery stools.

3. Mixed IBS (IBS-M): Symptoms alternate between constipation and diarrhea, with variable stool consistency.

4. Unsubtyped IBS (IBS-U): Symptoms do not fit into the above categories or shift between subtypes over time.

Diagnostic Challenges and Considerations:

While the Rome IV criteria provide a valuable framework for diagnosing IBS, there are certain challenges and considerations to be aware of:

Overlapping Symptoms: Some symptoms of IBS, such as abdominal pain and altered bowel habits, can overlap with other gastrointestinal disorders, necessitating thorough evaluation and differential diagnosis.

Subtypes of IBS: IBS can manifest with varying symptom patterns, including constipation-predominant (IBS-C), diarrhea-predominant (IBS-D), mixed (IBS-M), and unsubtyped (IBS-U) presentations. Healthcare providers should consider the predominant bowel habits and stool consistency when subtyping IBS for optimal management.

Exclusion of Organic Disorders: It is essential to exclude other organic gastrointestinal disorders that may mimic IBS, such as inflammatory bowel disease, celiac disease, and colorectal cancer, through appropriate diagnostic testing and evaluation.

Subtypes of IBS:

1. IBS with Constipation (IBS-C): IBS-C is characterized by predominant symptoms of constipation, including infrequent bowel movements, straining during defecation, and hard or lumpy stools. Individuals with IBS-C may experience abdominal discomfort or pain relieved by bowel movements, along with a sense of incomplete evacuation. Dietary factors, such as low fiber intake, dehydration, and sedentary lifestyle, may exacerbate constipation symptoms in IBS-C.

2. IBS with Diarrhea (IBS-D): IBS-D is characterized by predominant symptoms of diarrhea, including frequent bowel movements, urgency, and loose or watery stools. Abdominal pain or discomfort may be present and is often associated with bowel movements. Triggers for diarrhea in IBS-D may include certain foods, stress, or gastrointestinal infections. Individuals with IBS-D may also experience bloating and abdominal distension, albeit to a lesser extent than in IBS-C.

3. Mixed IBS (IBS-M): IBS-M is characterized by alternating or mixed symptoms of constipation and diarrhea, with variable stool consistency and frequency. Individuals with IBS-M may experience periods of constipation followed by episodes of diarrhea or vice versa. The fluctuating nature of symptoms in IBS-M can pose challenges in diagnosis and management, requiring a tailored approach that addresses both constipation and diarrhea symptoms.

4. Unsubtyped IBS (IBS-U): IBS-U refers to cases where symptoms do not fit into the above subtypes or where symptoms shift between subtypes over time. Individuals with IBS-U may experience a combination of constipation, diarrhea, and mixed symptoms, making it challenging to classify their condition into a specific subtype. Diagnostic evaluation and management of IBS-U should focus on addressing individual symptom patterns and underlying pathophysiological mechanisms.

Diagnostic Considerations:

Subtyping of IBS relies on a comprehensive assessment of symptom patterns, bowel habits, and stool consistency. Healthcare providers should elicit a detailed medical history, including the frequency and severity of bowel movements, associated symptoms (e.g., abdominal pain, bloating), and potential triggers (e.g., dietary factors, stress). Symptom diaries or bowel movement charts can aid in documenting symptom patterns over time and facilitating accurate subtyping of IBS.

In addition to clinical evaluation, diagnostic tests may be performed to rule out other gastrointestinal disorders and assess for comorbidities, such as inflammatory bowel disease, celiac disease, or gastrointestinal infections. Laboratory investigations, imaging studies, and endoscopic procedures may be indicated based on clinical suspicion and individual patient characteristics.

Therapeutic Implications:

Subtyping of IBS informs the selection of appropriate treatment strategies tailored to individual symptom profiles and patient preferences. Management of IBS subtypes may include:

- IBS-C: Dietary modifications (e.g., increased fiber intake, adequate hydration), laxatives (e.g., osmotic laxatives, stimulant laxatives), and prosecretory agents (e.g., lubiprostone, linaclotide).

- IBS-D: Dietary modifications (e.g., low-FODMAP diet), antidiarrheal medications (e.g., loperamide), bile acid sequestrants (e.g., cholestyramine), and gut-targeted therapies (e.g., rifaximin).

- IBS-M: Individualized treatment regimens addressing both constipation and diarrhea symptoms, such as combination therapies or alternating treatment approaches.

- IBS-U: Symptom-based management focusing on addressing individual symptom patterns and triggers, including dietary modifications, pharmacotherapy, and lifestyle interventions.

Differential diagnosis of IBS

- Inflammatory Bowel Disease (IBD): Inflammatory Bowel Disease, including Crohn's disease and ulcerative colitis, presents with symptoms similar to IBS, such as abdominal pain, altered bowel habits, diarrhea, and bloating. However, IBD is characterized by chronic inflammation of the gastrointestinal tract, which can be detected through endoscopic and histologic findings. Imaging studies, such as colonoscopy, computed tomography (CT) scans, and magnetic resonance imaging (MRI), aid in visualizing inflammation, mucosal lesions, and complications associated with IBD.
- Celiac Disease: Celiac Disease is an autoimmune disorder characterized by gluten intolerance, resulting in inflammation and damage to the small intestine. Symptoms of celiac disease may mimic those of IBS, including abdominal pain, bloating, diarrhea, and malabsorption. Serologic testing for specific antibodies (e.g., anti-tissue transglutaminase antibodies, anti-endomysial antibodies) and confirmatory small intestinal biopsy are essential for diagnosing celiac disease. Additionally, genetic testing for human leukocyte antigen (HLA) DQ2 and DQ8 alleles may aid in risk stratification for celiac disease.
- Small Intestinal Bacterial Overgrowth (SIBO): Small Intestinal Bacterial Overgrowth is characterized by an abnormal increase in bacterial colonization in the small intestine, leading to gastrointestinal symptoms such as bloating, abdominal pain, diarrhea, and malabsorption. Symptoms of SIBO can overlap with those of IBS, particularly in cases of IBS with diarrhea (IBS-D). Hydrogen breath testing, which measures the production of hydrogen and methane gases by colonic bacteria after ingestion of specific substrates (e.g., lactulose, glucose), is commonly used to diagnose SIBO.
- Functional Dyspepsia: Functional Dyspepsia is a common functional gastrointestinal disorder characterized by symptoms such as early satiety, postprandial fullness, epigastric pain, and bloating. While the predominant symptoms of functional dyspepsia differ from those of IBS, there is significant overlap, particularly in individuals with mixed upper and lower gastrointestinal symptoms. Clinical evaluation, including upper endoscopy and gastric emptying studies, may be performed to differentiate between functional dyspepsia and IBS.
- Colon Cancer: Colon Cancer can present with symptoms similar to those of IBS, including abdominal pain, altered bowel habits, and rectal bleeding. While less common, colon cancer should be considered in the differential diagnosis of individuals with new-onset or alarm symptoms suggestive of organic gastrointestinal disorders. Diagnostic evaluation typically includes colonoscopy, fecal occult blood testing, and imaging studies (e.g., abdominal CT scan, magnetic resonance imaging) to visualize the colon and identify neoplastic lesions.

CHAPTER TWO:

What Are Fodmap?

FODMAPs, which stands for Fermentable Oligosaccharides, Disaccharides, Monosaccharides, and Polyols, are a group of short-chain carbohydrates and sugar alcohols found in various foods. These compounds are poorly absorbed in the small intestine and can ferment in the colon, leading to gas production, bloating, abdominal discomfort, and altered bowel habits in susceptible individuals, particularly those with Irritable Bowel Syndrome (IBS) or other functional gastrointestinal disorders.

1. Fermentable Oligosaccharides: This category includes fructans and galacto-oligosaccharides (GOS). Fructans are present in foods such as wheat, onions, garlic, and certain fruits and vegetables, while GOS are found in legumes, lentils, and certain grains.

2. Disaccharides: The main disaccharide of concern is lactose, which is found in dairy products such as milk, yogurt, and soft cheeses. Lactose intolerance, caused by deficient lactase enzyme activity, can lead to gastrointestinal symptoms in individuals who are unable to digest lactose effectively.

3. Monosaccharides: The primary monosaccharide involved in the FODMAP group is excess fructose. Foods high in excess fructose include certain fruits (e.g., apples, pears, mangoes, watermelon), honey, and high-fructose corn syrup. Excess fructose absorption may be impaired in some individuals, leading to symptoms of bloating and discomfort.

4. Polyols: Polyols, also known as sugar alcohols, include sorbitol, mannitol, xylitol, and maltitol. These compounds are found naturally in certain fruits (e.g., apples, cherries, pears) and vegetables (e.g., cauliflower, mushrooms), as well as in artificially sweetened products such as sugar-free gum and candies. Polyols can have laxative effects and may exacerbate gastrointestinal symptoms in susceptible individuals.

Low-FODMAP Diet:

A low-FODMAP diet involves restricting the intake of foods high in FODMAPs and gradually reintroducing them to identify individual triggers and tolerances. The low-FODMAP diet is typically divided into three phases:

1. Elimination Phase: During this phase, high-FODMAP foods are eliminated from the diet for a specified period (usually 2-6 weeks) to reduce gastrointestinal symptoms and establish baseline symptom control.

2. Reintroduction Phase: Following the elimination phase, FODMAP-containing foods are systematically reintroduced in small quantities to identify specific triggers and determine individual tolerance levels. This phase involves careful monitoring of symptoms and may require guidance from a registered dietitian or healthcare provider.

3. Maintenance Phase: Once trigger foods have been identified, individuals can transition to a modified low-FODMAP diet that includes foods tolerated well without exacerbating symptoms. The goal is to achieve long-term symptom management while maintaining a balanced and varied diet.

Low-FODMAP Foods:

Low-FODMAP foods are well-tolerated alternatives that can be included in a low-FODMAP diet. While individual tolerance may vary, common low-FODMAP foods include:

1. Proteins: Meat, poultry, fish, eggs, tofu, tempeh, and lactose-free dairy products (e.g., lactose-free milk, hard cheeses).

2. Grains: Rice, oats, quinoa, gluten-free bread, pasta, and cereals made from corn or rice.

3. Fruits: Berries (e.g., strawberries, blueberries, raspberries), citrus fruits (e.g., oranges, lemons), bananas (ripe), grapes, and pineapple.

4. Vegetables: Leafy greens (e.g., spinach, kale, lettuce), carrots, cucumbers, bell peppers, zucchini, potatoes (white), and tomatoes (ripe).

5. Nuts and Seeds: Almonds (limited quantity), walnuts, macadamia nuts, pumpkin seeds, and sunflower seeds.

6. Fats and Oils: Olive oil, coconut oil, sesame oil, and avocado oil.

1. **Vegetables:**

   - Bell peppers (red, yellow, green)

   - Carrots

   - Cucumbers

   - Eggplant

   - Lettuce (e.g., iceberg, romaine)

   - Zucchini

   - Spinach

   - Kale

   - Swiss chard

   - Green beans

   - Bok choy

   - Alfalfa sprouts

2. **Fruits (in moderation and based on individual tolerance):**

   - Strawberries

   - Blueberries

   - Raspberries

- Oranges

- Pineapple

- Kiwi

- Cantaloupe

- Grapes

- Honeydew melon

- Bananas (underripe)

- Papaya

3. **Grains and Cereals:**

- Quinoa

- Rice (white, brown)

- Oats (certified gluten-free)

- Polenta (cornmeal)

- Buckwheat

- Millet

- Sorghum

- Corn (maize)

- Gluten-free breads and cereals made with low-FODMAP grains and flours

4. **Legumes and Pulses (in small portions, well-cooked, and based on individual tolerance):**

- Lentils (canned and rinsed)

- Chickpeas (canned and rinsed)

- Firm tofu (drained)

- Tempeh

- Edamame (shelled)

- Canned beans such as black beans, kidney beans, and navy beans (rinsed)

5. **Nuts and Seeds (in moderation and based on individual tolerance):**

- Almonds (serving size: up to 10 nuts)

- Walnuts (serving size: up to 10 halves)

- Pecans (serving size: up to 10 halves)

- Macadamia nuts (serving size: up to 20 nuts)

- Pumpkin seeds (serving size: up to 2 tablespoons)

- Sunflower seeds (serving size: up to 2 tablespoons)

- Chia seeds (serving size: up to 2 tablespoons)

- Flaxseeds (serving size: up to 2 tablespoons)

6. **Other Sources:**

- Coconut (shredded, unsweetened)

- Unsweetened coconut milk (in moderation)

- Unsweetened cocoa powder

- Seaweed (e.g., nori, kombu)

- Psyllium husk (as a fiber supplement, in moderation)

Low-FODMAP Sources of Protein

1. **Animal Proteins:**

   - Beef (e.g., steak, ground beef)

   - Chicken (e.g., breast, thigh)

   - Turkey (e.g., breast, ground)

   - Pork (e.g., tenderloin, chops)

   - Lamb

   - Fish (e.g., salmon, cod, trout, tuna, halibut)

   - Shellfish (e.g., shrimp, crab, lobster)

   - Eggs (whole eggs, egg whites)

2. **Plant-Based Proteins:**

   - Firm tofu (drained)

   - Tempeh

   - Edamame (shelled)

- Quinoa

- Firm or extra-firm tofu (drained)

- Tempeh

- Edamame (shelled)

- Chia seeds (in moderation)

- Flaxseeds (in moderation)

- Pumpkin seeds (in moderation)

- Sunflower seeds (in moderation)

- Hemp seeds (in moderation)

- Sesame seeds (in moderation)

- Pea protein powder (check ingredients for added FODMAPs)

3. **Dairy and Dairy Alternatives:**

- Lactose-free cow's milk (e.g., lactose-free cow's milk, lactose-free yogurt, lactose-free cheese)

- Hard cheeses (e.g., cheddar, Swiss, Parmesan)

- Lactose-free yogurt made from cow's milk or non-dairy alternatives (e.g., almond milk yogurt, coconut milk yogurt, lactose-free yogurt)

- Lactose-free cottage cheese

- Lactose-free kefir

- Almond milk (unsweetened)

- Coconut milk (unsweetened)

- Rice milk (unsweetened)

- Hemp milk (unsweetened)

- Oat milk (unsweetened)

4. **Nuts and Seeds (in moderation):**

- Almonds (serving size: up to 10 nuts)

- Walnuts (serving size: up to 10 halves)

- Pecans (serving size: up to 10 halves)

- Macadamia nuts (serving size: up to 20 nuts)

- Pumpkin seeds (serving size: up to 2 tablespoons)

- Sunflower seeds (serving size: up to 2 tablespoons)

- Chia seeds (serving size: up to 2 tablespoons)

- Flaxseeds (serving size: up to 2 tablespoons)

Low-FODMAP Sources of Calcium

1. **Lactose-Free Dairy Products:**

- Lactose-free cow's milk

- Lactose-free yogurt (plain or flavored)

- Lactose-free cheese (e.g., cheddar, Swiss, mozzarella)

- Lactose-free cottage cheese

2. **Non-Dairy Sources:**

- Almond milk (unsweetened)

- Coconut milk (unsweetened)

- Rice milk (unsweetened)

- Hemp milk (unsweetened)

- Oat milk (unsweetened)

- Calcium-fortified orange juice (check label for FODMAP content)

- Calcium-fortified non-dairy milk alternatives (e.g., almond milk, coconut milk, hemp milk)

3. **Green Leafy Vegetables:**

- Bok choy

- Kale

- Collard greens

- Turnip greens

- Swiss chard

- Spinach (in small portions)

4. **Canned Fish with Bones:**

- Canned salmon with bones

- Canned sardines with bones

5. **Firm Tofu:**

    - Firm tofu is a good source of calcium and can be used in various dishes such as stir-fries, soups, and salads.

6. **Fortified Foods:**

    - Some cereals, breads, and other grain products are fortified with calcium. Check the labels to ensure they are low in FODMAPs

Low FODMAO Pantry

1. **Grains and Cereals:**

    - Rice (white, brown)

    - Quinoa

    - Oats (certified gluten-free)

    - Polenta (cornmeal)

    - Buckwheat

    - Millet

    - Sorghum

    - Corn (maize)

    - Gluten-free pasta made from rice, quinoa, or corn

2. **Flours and Baking Ingredients:**

- Gluten-free all-purpose flour blends (rice flour, potato starch, tapioca starch)

- Cornstarch

- Potato starch

- Baking powder (check for wheat-based ingredients)

- Baking soda

- Xanthan gum (as a gluten-free binder)

3. **Canned and Jarred Goods:**

- Canned tomatoes (plain, no added garlic or onion)

- Canned vegetables (e.g., carrots, green beans, corn)

- Canned fruit (in natural juice, no added high-FODMAP sweeteners)

- Tomato paste (check for added garlic or onion)

- Low-FODMAP pasta sauce (check labels for garlic and onion content)

- Olives (pitted, no added garlic or onion)

4. **Proteins:**

- Canned tuna (packed in water)

- Canned salmon (with bones)

- Canned chicken (in water)

- Canned beans (lentils, chickpeas) - in moderation and rinsed well

- Nut butters (e.g., peanut butter, almond butter)

- Seeds (e.g., pumpkin seeds, sunflower seeds)

5. **Condiments and Sauces:**

- Low-FODMAP salad dressings (e.g., vinaigrettes made with olive oil and vinegar)

- Mayonnaise (check for added high-FODMAP ingredients)

- Mustard (check for added garlic or onion)

- Vinegars (e.g., white wine vinegar, apple cider vinegar)

- Soy sauce (gluten-free)

- Fish sauce (check for added high-FODMAP ingredients)

6. **Herbs and Spices:**

- Salt

- Pepper

- Dried herbs (e.g., oregano, basil, thyme)

- Spices (e.g., cumin, paprika, turmeric)

- Spice blends (check for added high-FODMAP ingredients)

7. **Oils and Fats:**

- Olive oil

- Coconut oil

- Vegetable oil

- Ghee (clarified butter)

- Butter (check for lactose content)

8. **Snacks and Treats:**

   - Rice cakes

   - Popcorn (plain, no added flavors)

   - Dark chocolate (in moderation)

   - Rice crackers

   - Potato chips (plain, no added flavors)

9. **Beverages:**

   - Water

   - Herbal teas (e.g., peppermint, chamomile)

   - Coffee (in moderation)

   - Tea (black, green)

10. **Miscellaneous:**

    - Low-FODMAP protein bars (check labels for high-FODMAP ingredients)

    - Gluten-free oats for baking (certified gluten-free)

    - Low-FODMAP sweeteners (e.g., maple syrup, glucose, stevia)

- Rice paper wraps (for making spring rolls)

- Gluten-free soy sauce alternatives (e.g., tamari, coconut aminos)

Practical Considerations:

When adopting a low-FODMAP diet, it is essential to:

- Consult with a registered dietitian or healthcare provider to ensure proper guidance and supervision throughout the dietary intervention.

- Keep a food diary to track symptoms and monitor responses to specific foods during the elimination and reintroduction phases.

- Read food labels carefully to identify hidden sources of FODMAPs in processed foods and condiments.

- Plan meals and snacks in advance to ensure adequate nutrient intake and variety while adhering to the low-FODMAP guidelines.

- Be mindful of potential psychological and social impacts of dietary restrictions and seek support from family, friends, and support groups when neede

Identifying Trigger Foods

Identifying trigger foods is a crucial aspect of managing Irritable Bowel Syndrome (IBS) and other gastrointestinal disorders. By recognizing specific foods that exacerbate symptoms, individuals can make informed dietary choices to alleviate discomfort and improve quality of life. Here's a guide on how to identify trigger foods:

1. Keep a Food Diary: Start by keeping a detailed food diary to track your daily dietary intake and any associated symptoms. Record not only what you eat but also portion sizes, meal times, and symptom onset, duration, and severity. This information will provide valuable insights into potential trigger foods and their impact on your digestive health.

2. Note Symptom Patterns: Pay close attention to patterns or correlations between certain foods and gastrointestinal symptoms. Common symptoms associated with trigger foods include abdominal pain, bloating, gas, diarrhea, constipation, and heartburn. Look for consistent patterns of symptom exacerbation following the consumption of specific foods or food groups.

3. Follow the Low-FODMAP Diet: Consider following a low-FODMAP diet, which involves eliminating high-FODMAP foods from your diet for a period of time and then systematically reintroducing them to identify individual triggers. FODMAPs are fermentable carbohydrates and sugar alcohols found in certain foods that can exacerbate symptoms in individuals with IBS. By following a structured approach to eliminating and reintroducing FODMAPs, you can identify specific trigger foods and their tolerance levels.

4. Gradually Reintroduce Foods: Once you have completed the elimination phase of the low-FODMAP diet, gradually reintroduce one high-FODMAP food at a time in small quantities. Monitor your symptoms closely for any adverse reactions or exacerbation of gastrointestinal symptoms. Keep track of which foods trigger symptoms and the severity of your response.

5. Consider Other Potential Triggers: In addition to FODMAPs, other dietary factors such as caffeine, spicy foods, fatty foods, artificial sweeteners, and alcohol can contribute to gastrointestinal symptoms in some individuals. Pay attention to these factors and their impact on your digestive health. It may be helpful to eliminate or reduce these potential triggers while assessing their effect on your symptoms.

6. Seek Professional Guidance: Consult with a registered dietitian or healthcare provider who specializes in gastrointestinal disorders for personalized guidance and support in identifying trigger foods and implementing dietary modifications. They can help you develop a tailored dietary plan, provide education on label reading and food preparation, and offer strategies for managing symptoms effectively.

Low-FODMAP Ingredients

Stocking your kitchen with low-FODMAP ingredients is essential for managing Irritable Bowel Syndrome (IBS) symptoms while following a low-FODMAP diet. Here's a comprehensive list of low-FODMAP ingredients to include in your pantry, refrigerator, and freezer:

Grains and Cereals:

- Rice (white, brown, jasmine, basmati)

- Quinoa

- Oats (certified gluten-free)

- Cornmeal (polenta)

- Millet

- Sorghum

- Buckwheat

- Gluten-free pasta (made from rice, quinoa, or corn)

Flours and Baking Ingredients:

- Gluten-free all-purpose flour blends (rice flour, potato starch, tapioca starch)

- Cornstarch

- Potato starch

- Baking powder (check for wheat-based ingredients)

- Baking soda

- Xanthan gum (as a gluten-free binder)

Fruits (in moderation):

- Strawberries

- Blueberries

- Raspberries

- Oranges

- Kiwi

- Pineapple

- Grapes

- Honeydew melon

- Cantaloupe

- Bananas (unripe)

Vegetables (in moderation):

- Bell peppers (red, yellow, green)

- Carrots

- Cucumbers

- Eggplant

- Lettuce (e.g., iceberg, romaine)

- Zucchini

- Spinach

- Kale

- Swiss chard

- Green beans

- Bok choy

- Alfalfa sprouts

Proteins:

- Beef (lean cuts)

- Chicken (skinless breast)

- Turkey (skinless breast)

- Pork (tenderloin)

- Fish (e.g., salmon, cod, trout, tuna, halibut)

- Shellfish (e.g., shrimp, crab, lobster)

- Eggs (whole eggs, egg whites)

- Firm tofu (drained)

- Tempeh

- Edamame (shelled)

- Canned tuna (in water)

- Canned salmon (with bones)

Dairy and Dairy Alternatives:

- Lactose-free cow's milk

- Lactose-free yogurt (plain or flavored)

- Lactose-free cheese (e.g., cheddar, Swiss, mozzarella)

- Lactose-free cottage cheese

- Almond milk (unsweetened)

- Coconut milk (unsweetened)

- Rice milk (unsweetened)

- Hemp milk (unsweetened)

- Oat milk (unsweetened)

Nuts and Seeds (in moderation):

- Almonds (serving size: up to 10 nuts)

- Walnuts (serving size: up to 10 halves)

- Pecans (serving size: up to 10 halves)

- Macadamia nuts (serving size: up to 20 nuts)

- Pumpkin seeds (serving size: up to 2 tablespoons)

- Sunflower seeds (serving size: up to 2 tablespoons)

* Chia seeds (serving size: up to 2 tablespoons)

* Flaxseeds (serving size: up to 2 tablespoons)

Oils and Fats:

* Olive oil

* Coconut oil

* Vegetable oil

* Ghee (clarified butter)

* Butter (check for lactose content)

Herbs and Spices:

* Salt

* Pepper

* Dried herbs (e.g., oregano, basil, thyme)

* Spices (e.g., cumin, paprika, turmeric)

* Spice blends (check for high-FODMAP ingredients)

Condiments and Sauces:

* Low-FODMAP salad dressings (e.g., vinaigrettes made with olive oil and vinegar)

* Mayonnaise (check for high-FODMAP ingredients)

* Mustard (check for high-FODMAP ingredients)

- Vinegars (e.g., white wine vinegar, apple cider vinegar)

- Soy sauce (gluten-free)

- Fish sauce (check for high-FODMAP ingredients)

Miscellaneous:

- Rice cakes

- Popcorn (plain, no added flavors)

- Dark chocolate (in moderation)

- Gluten-free soy sauce alternatives (e.g., tamari, coconut aminos)

- Low-FODMAP protein bars (check labels for high-FODMAP ingredients)

- Gluten-free oats for baking (certified gluten-free)

- Low-FODMAP sweeteners (e.g., maple syrup, glucose, stevia)

- Rice paper wraps (for making spring rolls)

Creating a Balanced Meal Plan for IBS

Creating a balanced meal plan for Irritable Bowel Syndrome (IBS) involves selecting foods that are well-tolerated, nutrient-rich, and supportive of gastrointestinal health. Here's a guide to help you create a balanced meal plan tailored to managing IBS symptoms:

1. **Focus on Low-FODMAP Foods:** Base your meals around low-FODMAP foods that are less likely to trigger gastrointestinal symptoms. Incorporate plenty of fruits, vegetables, proteins, and grains that are low in fermentable carbohydrates and sugar alcohols.

2. **Include Lean Proteins:** Choose lean sources of protein such as poultry, fish, eggs, tofu, and tempeh. These protein sources are generally well-tolerated and provide essential nutrients without exacerbating IBS symptoms.

3. **Incorporate Low-FODMAP Fruits and Vegetables:** Include a variety of low-FODMAP fruits and vegetables in your meals to ensure adequate fiber intake and micronutrient content. Opt for options such as spinach, kale, carrots, cucumbers, strawberries, blueberries, oranges, and grapes.

4. **Choose Gluten-Free Grains:** If you find that gluten exacerbates your IBS symptoms, choose gluten-free grains such as rice, quinoa, oats, and corn. These grains are naturally low in FODMAPs and provide fiber, vitamins, and minerals to support digestive health.

5. **Include Healthy Fats:** Incorporate sources of healthy fats into your meals, such as olive oil, avocado, nuts, and seeds. These fats provide essential fatty acids and promote satiety without causing digestive discomfort.

6. **Limit Trigger Foods:** Identify and limit or avoid trigger foods that exacerbate your IBS symptoms. Common trigger foods include high-FODMAP foods, spicy foods, fatty foods, caffeine, alcohol, and artificial sweeteners.

7. **Practice Portion Control:** Pay attention to portion sizes to prevent overeating, which can contribute to gastrointestinal discomfort. Eating smaller, more frequent meals throughout the day may be beneficial for some individuals with IBS.

8. **Stay Hydrated:** Drink plenty of water throughout the day to stay hydrated and support healthy digestion. Aim for at least 8-10 cups of water per day, and limit or avoid carbonated beverages and drinks with high caffeine content.

Sample Balanced Meal Plan for IBS:

Breakfast:

- Oatmeal made with lactose-free milk, topped with strawberries and a tablespoon of almond butter.

- Green tea or peppermint tea.

Lunch:

- Grilled chicken breast with quinoa and steamed carrots and zucchini.

- Spinach salad with cucumber, cherry tomatoes, and a light olive oil vinaigrette.

Snack:

- Rice cakes with peanut butter or a handful of mixed nuts (e.g., almonds, walnuts).

- Orange slices or grapes.

Dinner:

- Baked salmon with roasted potatoes and green beans.

- Quinoa salad with diced bell peppers, cucumber, and a lemon-herb dressing.

Evening Snack (if needed):

- Greek yogurt with lactose-free yogurt topped with low-FODMAP granola or a banana.

Medications for IBS

Medications for Irritable Bowel Syndrome (IBS) aim to alleviate symptoms and improve overall quality of life for individuals affected by this chronic gastrointestinal disorder. Treatment strategies may vary depending on the predominant symptoms (constipation, diarrhea, or mixed) and the severity of symptoms. Here's an overview of common medications used to manage IBS:

1. **Antispasmodics:** Antispasmodic medications such as hyoscyamine (Levsin), dicyclomine (Bentyl), and peppermint oil (enteric-coated capsules) can help reduce abdominal pain and cramping by relaxing smooth muscles in the gastrointestinal tract. These medications are particularly useful for individuals with IBS-D or IBS-M.

2. **Antidiarrheal Agents:** For individuals with diarrhea-predominant IBS (IBS-D), antidiarrheal medications such as loperamide (Imodium) can help reduce stool frequency and improve stool consistency. Loperamide works by slowing down intestinal motility and increasing water absorption in the colon.

3. **Laxatives:** Laxative medications may be recommended for individuals with constipation-predominant IBS (IBS-C) to alleviate symptoms of constipation and promote regular bowel movements. Options include osmotic laxatives (e.g., polyethylene glycol, lactulose), stimulant laxatives (e.g., bisacodyl, senna), and lubiprostone (Amitiza), which increases fluid secretion in the intestines.

4. **Serotonin Modulators:** Serotonin plays a key role in regulating gastrointestinal motility and sensation. Medications that modulate serotonin levels in the gut, such as selective serotonin reuptake inhibitors (SSRIs) and serotonin-norepinephrine reuptake inhibitors (SNRIs), may be prescribed to alleviate symptoms of IBS, particularly abdominal pain and discomfort.

5. **Tricyclic Antidepressants (TCAs):** TCAs, such as amitriptyline and nortriptyline, are sometimes used off-label to treat symptoms of IBS, including abdominal pain, bloating, and altered bowel habits. TCAs can help modulate pain perception and improve gut

motility, although their use may be limited by side effects such as drowsiness and dry mouth.

6. **Bile Acid Sequestrants:** Bile acid sequestrants, such as cholestyramine and colesevelam, may be prescribed for individuals with bile acid malabsorption or bile acid diarrhea, which can occur in some cases of IBS-D. These medications bind to bile acids in the intestine, reducing bile acid concentration and improving symptoms.

7. **Antidepressants:** Certain antidepressant medications, such as selective serotonin reuptake inhibitors (SSRIs) and serotonin-norepinephrine reuptake inhibitors (SNRIs), may be prescribed to manage symptoms of IBS, particularly when associated with psychological comorbidities such as anxiety and depression. These medications can help modulate pain perception and improve mood, which may indirectly benefit gastrointestinal symptoms.

8. **Probiotics:** Probiotic supplements containing beneficial bacteria strains, such as Lactobacillus and Bifidobacterium species, may be used to restore gut microbiota balance and alleviate symptoms of IBS, particularly bloating and abdominal discomfort. However, the evidence supporting the efficacy of probiotics in IBS is mixed, and more research is needed to determine their optimal use.

It's essential to consult with a healthcare provider to determine the most appropriate medication regimen based on your individual symptoms, medical history, and treatment goals. Additionally, lifestyle modifications, dietary changes, stress management techniques, and other non-pharmacological approaches may complement medication therapy in managing IBS symptoms effectively.

Psychological interventions for IBS

1. **Cognitive Behavioral Therapy (CBT):** CBT is a structured, evidence-based psychotherapy approach that focuses on identifying and challenging negative thought patterns and maladaptive behaviors. In the context of IBS, CBT helps individuals develop coping skills to manage stress, anxiety, and symptoms related to IBS. CBT techniques may include cognitive restructuring, relaxation training, stress management, and behavioral activation.

2. **Hypnotherapy:** Hypnotherapy involves inducing a relaxed state of consciousness (hypnosis) to promote relaxation, focus attention, and facilitate positive therapeutic suggestions. Hypnotherapy has been shown to be effective in reducing gastrointestinal symptoms, including abdominal pain, bloating, and bowel dysfunction, in individuals with IBS. It may also help alleviate psychological distress and improve overall well-being.

3. **Mindfulness-Based Stress Reduction (MBSR):** MBSR is a structured mindfulness meditation program that teaches individuals to cultivate present-moment awareness, non-judgmental acceptance, and self-compassion. MBSR practices, such as mindfulness meditation, body scan, and mindful movement, can help individuals with IBS develop greater resilience to stress, reduce anxiety, and improve their ability to cope with gastrointestinal symptoms.

4. **Relaxation Techniques:** Various relaxation techniques, such as progressive muscle relaxation, deep breathing exercises, guided imagery, and autogenic training, can promote relaxation and alleviate tension in the body and mind. These techniques can be incorporated into daily routines to reduce stress, manage anxiety, and mitigate symptoms of IBS.

5. **Biofeedback:** Biofeedback is a therapeutic technique that utilizes electronic monitoring devices to provide real-time feedback on physiological processes, such as heart rate variability, muscle tension, and skin temperature. Biofeedback training helps individuals with IBS gain awareness and control over physiological responses associated with stress and gastrointestinal symptoms, leading to symptom improvement and enhanced self-regulation.

6. **Stress Management Programs:** Structured stress management programs, such as stress reduction workshops, relaxation training, and coping skills training, can provide education, support, and practical strategies for managing stress and its impact on IBS symptoms. These programs often incorporate elements of CBT, mindfulness, and relaxation techniques to empower individuals with IBS to effectively cope with stressors in their lives.

7. **Support Groups and Peer Counseling:** Participating in support groups, either in-person or online, can provide a sense of community, validation, and emotional support for individuals with IBS. Peer counseling and shared experiences can help reduce feelings of isolation, foster coping skills, and promote self-care among individuals living with IBS.

CHAPTER THREE:

Managing IBS-related anxiety and Emotional Eating

Managing anxiety and emotional eating in the context of Irritable Bowel Syndrome (IBS) is crucial for improving overall well-being and symptom management. Anxiety and stress can exacerbate IBS symptoms, while emotional eating may lead to dietary choices that trigger gastrointestinal distress. Here are some strategies for managing IBS-related anxiety and emotional eating:

1. **Stress Reduction Techniques:**

   - Practice relaxation techniques such as deep breathing, progressive muscle relaxation, mindfulness meditation, and guided imagery to reduce stress and promote relaxation. Regular practice of these techniques can help alleviate anxiety and calm the nervous system, which may in turn improve IBS symptoms.

   - Engage in activities that promote relaxation and stress relief, such as yoga, tai chi, gentle exercise, spending time in nature, listening to music, or engaging in hobbies that you enjoy.

2. **Cognitive Behavioral Therapy (CBT):**

   - Consider undergoing cognitive behavioral therapy (CBT) with a qualified therapist who specializes in gastrointestinal disorders. CBT can help you identify and challenge negative thought patterns, develop coping strategies for managing anxiety and stress, and address maladaptive behaviors such as emotional eating.

   - Learn cognitive restructuring techniques to challenge irrational beliefs and distorted thinking patterns that contribute to anxiety and emotional eating. Replace negative thoughts with more realistic and adaptive ones to reduce emotional distress.

3. **Mindfulness-Based Practices:**

   - Practice mindfulness-based interventions such as mindfulness meditation, mindful eating, and body scan exercises. Mindfulness can help you cultivate present-moment awareness, non-judgmental acceptance, and self-compassion, which can reduce emotional reactivity and promote healthier eating habits.

   - Use mindfulness techniques to tune into your body's hunger and fullness cues, as well as your emotional state, before eating. This can help you distinguish between physical hunger and emotional hunger, and make more mindful choices about when and what to eat.

4. **Healthy Coping Strategies:**

- Identify alternative coping strategies for managing stress and emotional distress that do not involve food. Practice self-care activities such as journaling, taking a warm bath, practicing relaxation exercises, or seeking social support from friends and family.

- Engage in regular physical activity, which can help reduce stress, improve mood, and promote overall well-being. Find activities that you enjoy and incorporate them into your daily routine to support your mental and physical health.

5. **Nutrition Education:**

- Seek guidance from a registered dietitian or nutritionist who specializes in gastrointestinal health to learn about the impact of diet on IBS symptoms and strategies for managing emotional eating. Educate yourself about low-FODMAP foods, portion control, balanced nutrition, and mindful eating practices.

- Work with a dietitian to develop a personalized meal plan that meets your nutritional needs, supports digestive health, and minimizes triggers for IBS symptoms. Focus on incorporating whole, unprocessed foods, fiber-rich fruits and vegetables, lean proteins, and healthy fats into your diet.

6. **Seek Professional Support:**

- If anxiety, stress, or emotional eating significantly impact your quality of life and ability to manage IBS symptoms, consider seeking support from a mental health professional, such as a psychologist or counselor. Therapy can provide a safe and supportive environment to explore and address underlying emotional issues and develop coping skills for managing anxiety and emotional eating.

Probiotics play a significant role in supporting gut health by promoting a balanced microbiota, enhancing immune function, and modulating gastrointestinal function. The term "probiotic" refers to live microorganisms that, when administered in adequate amounts, confer health benefits to the host. These beneficial bacteria can colonize the intestines, compete with harmful bacteria for nutrients and attachment sites, and produce compounds that support digestive health. Here's how probiotics contribute to gut health:

1. **Restoring Microbial Balance:** Probiotics help maintain a diverse and balanced gut microbiota, which is essential for proper digestion, nutrient absorption, and immune function. Factors such as antibiotic use, stress, diet, and illness can disrupt the microbial balance in the gut, leading to dysbiosis and gastrointestinal symptoms. Probiotic supplementation can help restore microbial balance and support overall gut health.

2. **Enhancing Immune Function:** The gut-associated lymphoid tissue (GALT) plays a crucial role in immune function and defense against pathogens in the gastrointestinal tract. Probiotics stimulate the production of immunoglobulins, cytokines, and other immune mediators that enhance the body's immune response and help protect against infections and inflammation. By strengthening the gut barrier and modulating immune function, probiotics contribute to a healthy gut and overall immune system.

3. **Modulating Gastrointestinal Function:** Probiotics exert various effects on gastrointestinal function, including regulating gut motility, reducing intestinal inflammation, and improving intestinal barrier function. Certain strains of probiotics can help alleviate symptoms of digestive disorders such as Irritable Bowel Syndrome (IBS), inflammatory bowel disease (IBD), diarrhea, and constipation by modulating gut physiology and reducing gut-related symptoms.

4. **Producing Beneficial Metabolites:** Probiotic bacteria produce a range of metabolites and bioactive compounds that contribute to gut health and overall well-being. These include short-chain fatty acids (SCFAs) such as acetate, propionate, and butyrate, which serve as energy sources for colonocytes, regulate immune function, and maintain intestinal barrier integrity. Probiotics can also produce antimicrobial peptides, vitamins, enzymes, and other bioactive molecules that support digestive health.

5. **Promoting Nutrient Absorption:** Probiotics can enhance nutrient absorption in the intestines by improving the breakdown and utilization of dietary nutrients such as carbohydrates, proteins, fats, vitamins, and minerals. By fermenting dietary fibers and complex carbohydrates, probiotics produce metabolites that promote nutrient absorption, enhance satiety, and support metabolic health.

6. **Supporting Mental Health:** Emerging research suggests a link between gut health and mental health, known as the gut-brain axis. Probiotics may exert beneficial effects on mood, cognition, and emotional well-being by modulating gut microbiota composition,

reducing inflammation, and influencing neurotransmitter signaling pathways. Probiotic supplementation has been shown to improve symptoms of anxiety, depression, and stress-related disorders in some studies.

Efficacy of Probiotics

The efficacy of probiotics in promoting health and managing various medical conditions has been extensively studied in scientific research. While the effects of probiotics can vary depending on factors such as the specific strains used, dosage, duration of use, and individual health status, evidence suggests that probiotics offer several potential health benefits. Here's an overview of the efficacy of probiotics based on research findings:

1. **Digestive Health:** Probiotics have been shown to be effective in improving digestive health by promoting gastrointestinal motility, regulating bowel habits, and alleviating symptoms of digestive disorders such as Irritable Bowel Syndrome (IBS), inflammatory bowel disease (IBD), diarrhea, constipation, and gastroenteritis. Certain strains of probiotics, such as Lactobacillus rhamnosus GG and Saccharomyces boulardii, have demonstrated efficacy in reducing the duration and severity of acute infectious diarrhea and antibiotic-associated diarrhea.

2. **Immune Function:** Probiotics play a role in modulating immune function and enhancing the body's defense mechanisms against infections and inflammation. Research suggests that probiotics can stimulate the production of immunoglobulins, cytokines, and other immune mediators that help protect against respiratory infections, gastrointestinal infections, urinary tract infections, and allergic conditions. Probiotics may also reduce the risk of developing allergic diseases such as eczema and asthma in infants and children.

3. **Women's Health:** Probiotics have been investigated for their potential benefits in promoting women's health, particularly in preventing and managing urogenital infections such as bacterial vaginosis, yeast infections (vulvovaginal candidiasis), and urinary tract infections (UTIs). Certain strains of probiotics, such as Lactobacillus acidophilus and Lactobacillus rhamnosus GR-1, have been shown to help maintain vaginal microbial balance and reduce the recurrence of urogenital infections in women.

4. **Metabolic Health:** Probiotics may have beneficial effects on metabolic health by modulating lipid metabolism, glucose metabolism, and insulin sensitivity. Studies have suggested that certain strains of probiotics, such as Lactobacillus and Bifidobacterium species, can help reduce serum cholesterol levels, improve glycemic control, and reduce markers of inflammation and oxidative stress in individuals with metabolic syndrome, type 2 diabetes, and obesity.

5. **Mental Health:** Emerging research suggests a link between gut health and mental health, known as the gut-brain axis. Probiotics may exert beneficial effects on mood, cognition, and emotional well-being by modulating gut microbiota composition, reducing inflammation, and influencing neurotransmitter signaling pathways. Some studies have suggested that probiotic supplementation may help alleviate symptoms of anxiety, depression, and stress-related disorders, although further research is needed to establish definitive conclusions.

6. **Oral Health:** Probiotics have been investigated for their potential role in promoting oral health and preventing oral diseases such as dental caries (cavities) and periodontal disease (gum disease). Certain strains of probiotics, such as Lactobacillus reuteri and Lactobacillus paracasei, have been shown to inhibit the growth of cavity-causing bacteria, reduce plaque formation, and support gum health when used as adjuncts to oral hygiene measures.

Recommended Probiotic Strains

1. **Lactobacillus acidophilus (L. acidophilus):**

   - This probiotic strain is commonly found in yogurt and other fermented dairy products.

   - Benefits: L. acidophilus has been shown to support digestive health, promote immune function, and prevent or alleviate symptoms of diarrhea, lactose intolerance, and vaginal infections.

   - Applications: It may be helpful for individuals with digestive issues, immune system imbalances, or urogenital infections.

2. **Lactobacillus rhamnosus (L. rhamnosus):**

   - This versatile probiotic strain is well-studied and widely used in various probiotic formulations.

   - Benefits: L. rhamnosus has been shown to support gastrointestinal health, reduce symptoms of diarrhea, prevent urinary tract infections, and enhance immune function.

   - Applications: It may be beneficial for individuals with gastrointestinal disorders, antibiotic-associated diarrhea, urinary tract infections, or allergies.

3. **Bifidobacterium bifidum (B. bifidum):**

- This probiotic strain is naturally found in the human colon and is important for maintaining gut health.

- Benefits: B. bifidum helps support digestive health, regulate bowel movements, and reduce inflammation in the intestines.

- Applications: It may be beneficial for individuals with irritable bowel syndrome (IBS), inflammatory bowel disease (IBD), constipation, or allergies.

4. **Bifidobacterium lactis (B. lactis):**

- This probiotic strain is known for its resilience and ability to survive passage through the acidic environment of the stomach.

- Benefits: B. lactis has been shown to support digestive health, enhance immune function, and alleviate symptoms of diarrhea and constipation.

- Applications: It may be helpful for individuals with digestive disorders, immune system imbalances, or lactose intolerance.

5. **Saccharomyces boulardii:**

- Unlike bacterial probiotics, S. boulardii is a yeast probiotic that has been extensively studied for its health benefits.

- Benefits: S. boulardii helps support gastrointestinal health, reduce symptoms of diarrhea (including antibiotic-associated diarrhea and traveler's diarrhea), and prevent recurrent Clostridium difficile (C. diff) infections.

- Applications: It may be beneficial for individuals with acute diarrhea, antibiotic-associated diarrhea, or gastrointestinal infections.

6. **Lactobacillus plantarum:**

- This probiotic strain is known for its ability to survive in harsh environments and adhere to the intestinal lining.

- Benefits: L. plantarum has been shown to support digestive health, reduce inflammation, and promote immune function.

- Applications: It may be beneficial for individuals with gastrointestinal disorders, inflammatory conditions, or immune system imbalances.

Vitamin and Mineral Supplements:

Vitamin and mineral supplements can play a role in supporting overall health and well-being, including for individuals with Irritable Bowel Syndrome (IBS). While nutrient deficiencies are not typically a primary cause of IBS, certain vitamins and minerals may help alleviate symptoms or support gut health. Here's how some key nutrients and supplements may impact IBS:

1. **Fiber Supplements:** Soluble fiber supplements such as psyllium husk or methylcellulose may help improve bowel regularity and alleviate symptoms of constipation in individuals with IBS-C (constipation-predominant IBS). However, it's important to introduce fiber supplements gradually and increase fluid intake to prevent worsening of symptoms such as bloating or gas.

2. **Probiotic Supplements:** Probiotic supplements containing beneficial bacteria strains, such as Lactobacillus and Bifidobacterium species, may help restore gut microbiota balance and alleviate symptoms of IBS, particularly bloating and abdominal discomfort. While the evidence supporting the efficacy of probiotics in IBS is mixed, some individuals may benefit from probiotic supplementation.

3. **Vitamin D:** Adequate vitamin D levels are important for immune function, bone health, and overall well-being. Some studies suggest that vitamin D deficiency may be more common in individuals with IBS, although the relationship between vitamin D status and IBS symptoms is not fully understood. Maintaining adequate vitamin D levels through supplementation or sun exposure may be beneficial for some individuals with IBS.

4. **Magnesium:** Magnesium supplementation may help alleviate symptoms of constipation in individuals with IBS-C by promoting bowel motility and muscle relaxation. However, excessive magnesium intake can cause diarrhea and should be avoided in individuals with diarrhea-predominant IBS (IBS-D).

5. **Iron:** Iron deficiency anemia may occur in individuals with chronic gastrointestinal disorders such as IBS, particularly if there is underlying intestinal bleeding or malabsorption. Iron supplementation may be necessary to correct iron deficiency and prevent anemia, although it's important to monitor iron levels and consider the form of iron (e.g., ferrous sulfate vs. ferrous gluconate) to minimize gastrointestinal side effects.

Hydration and Impact on IBS:

Proper hydration is essential for maintaining overall health and well-being, including for individuals with Irritable Bowel Syndrome (IBS). Adequate fluid intake helps support digestion, regulate bowel function, and prevent dehydration, which can exacerbate symptoms of IBS. Here's how hydration can impact IBS:

1. **Maintaining Bowel Regularity:** Drinking enough fluids, particularly water, helps keep stools soft and promotes regular bowel movements. Adequate hydration can help prevent or alleviate symptoms of constipation in individuals with IBS-C (constipation-predominant IBS) by softening stools and easing their passage through the intestines.

2. **Preventing Dehydration:** Chronic diarrhea, a common symptom of IBS-D (diarrhea-predominant IBS), can lead to fluid loss and dehydration if not adequately managed. It's important for individuals with IBS-D to stay well-hydrated by drinking plenty of fluids throughout the day to replace lost fluids and electrolytes.

3. **Reducing Bloating and Discomfort:** Drinking fluids, especially non-caffeinated and non-carbonated beverages, can help alleviate bloating and discomfort in individuals with IBS. Avoiding excessive intake of carbonated beverages and caffeinated drinks, which can exacerbate bloating and gas, may also help reduce gastrointestinal symptoms.

4. **Choosing Hydrating Foods:** Consuming hydrating foods with high water content, such as fruits, vegetables, soups, and broths, can contribute to overall hydration and help maintain fluid balance in the body. Including hydrating foods in the diet can also provide essential nutrients, fiber, and antioxidants that support gut health and overall well-being.

5. **Monitoring Fluid Intake:** Pay attention to your body's thirst cues and drink water or other hydrating beverages regularly throughout the day. Aim to drink at least 8-10 cups (64-80 ounces) of fluids daily, or more if you have increased fluid needs due to factors such as exercise, hot weather, or illness.

6. **Limiting Trigger Beverages:** Certain beverages, such as alcohol, caffeinated drinks, and sugary sodas, may exacerbate symptoms of IBS in some individuals. It's important to be mindful of your beverage choices and limit or avoid beverages that trigger gastrointestinal symptoms or worsen hydration status.

Regular physical activity and exercise can have a positive impact on Irritable Bowel Syndrome (IBS) by helping to manage symptoms, reduce stress, improve overall well-being, and support digestive health. While the relationship between exercise and IBS is complex and may vary among individuals, incorporating regular exercise into your routine can offer several potential benefits:

1. **Improving Bowel Function:** Exercise can help regulate bowel function and alleviate symptoms of constipation or diarrhea in individuals with IBS. Physical activity stimulates bowel motility and promotes more regular and efficient movement of stool through the intestines, which may help prevent or relieve symptoms of gastrointestinal discomfort and irregularity.

2. **Reducing Stress and Anxiety:** Physical activity has been shown to reduce stress, anxiety, and depression, which are common triggers for IBS symptoms. Regular exercise releases endorphins and other neurotransmitters that promote feelings of well-being and relaxation, helping to alleviate psychological stress and improve mood.

3. **Promoting Weight Management:** Maintaining a healthy weight through regular exercise and physical activity can help reduce the severity of IBS symptoms, particularly in individuals with obesity or overweight. Exercise supports weight management by increasing energy expenditure, building lean muscle mass, and improving metabolic health, which may help alleviate symptoms such as abdominal pain, bloating, and discomfort.

4. **Enhancing Gut Health:** Exercise may have beneficial effects on gut microbiota composition and diversity, which play a crucial role in digestive health and immune function. Regular physical activity has been associated with a more diverse and balanced gut microbiota, reduced intestinal inflammation, and improved gut barrier function, all of which may contribute to symptom relief in individuals with IBS.

5. **Promoting Relaxation and Sleep:** Engaging in physical activity can promote relaxation and improve sleep quality, both of which are important for managing stress and supporting overall well-being in individuals with IBS. Regular exercise can help reduce insomnia, promote restful sleep, and enhance the body's ability to cope with stressors, which may in turn improve symptoms of IBS.

6. **Choosing Suitable Activities**: When incorporating exercise into your routine, choose activities that you enjoy and can comfortably participate in without exacerbating symptoms of IBS. Low-impact exercises such as walking, swimming, cycling, yoga, tai chi, and Pilates are generally well-tolerated and can be modified to suit individual fitness levels and preferences.

7. **Gradual Progression**: If you're new to exercise or have been inactive for a while, start slowly and gradually increase the intensity, duration, and frequency of your workouts

over time. Listen to your body and pay attention to how different types of exercise affect your symptoms, adjusting your routine as needed to find the right balance for you.

CHAPTER FOUR

Practical Cooking Tips and Recipes for IBS

BREAKFAST

Rice Porridge with Berries:

Prep Time: 15 minutes   **Servings:** 2-4

Ingredients:

• 1 cup white rice

• 2 cups lactose-free milk

• 1 teaspoon vanilla extract

• 1 tablespoon maple syrup (optional)

• 1 cup mixed berries (such as strawberries, blueberries, and raspberries)

• 2 tablespoons pumpkin seeds (optional, for topping)

Instructions:

1. Rinse the rice under cold water until the water runs clear. Drain well.

2. In a medium-sized saucepan, combine the rice and lactose-free milk. Bring to a boil over medium heat.

3. Once boiling, reduce the heat to low and simmer, stirring occasionally, for about 20-25 minutes, or until the rice is tender and the mixture has thickened to a porridge-like consistency.

4. Stir in the vanilla extract and maple syrup, if using.

5. Divide the rice porridge among serving bowls.

6. Top each bowl with a generous portion of mixed berries.

7. Sprinkle with pumpkin seeds, if desired.

8. Serve warm and enjoy!

Nutritional Values (Approximate, per serving):

Calories: 250-300 kcal | Protein: 8-10 grams | Fat: 4-6 grams | Saturated Fat: 1-2 grams | Carbohydrates: 45-50 grams | Dietary Fiber: 3-4 grams | Sugars: 10-12 grams

Bacon and Zucchini Crustless Quiche:

Prep Time: 15 minutes   **Servings**: 6-8

Ingredients:

- 6 slices bacon, chopped

- 1 medium zucchini, grated

- 1 cup cherry tomatoes, halved

- 1 cup shredded cheddar cheese

- 6 large eggs

- 1/2 cup lactose-free milk

- 1/4 teaspoon garlic powder

- Salt and pepper, to taste

- Fresh parsley, chopped, for garnish

Instructions:

1. Preheat your oven to 350°F (175°C). Grease a 9-inch pie dish.

2. In a skillet over medium heat, cook the chopped bacon until crispy. Remove from the skillet and drain on paper towels.

3. In the same skillet, add the grated zucchini and cook for 3-4 minutes until softened. Remove from heat and let cool slightly.

4. In a large bowl, whisk together the eggs, lactose-free milk, garlic powder, salt, and pepper.

5. Stir in the cooked bacon, grated zucchini, halved cherry tomatoes, and shredded cheddar cheese until well combined.

6. Pour the egg mixture into the prepared pie dish.

7. Bake in the preheated oven for 35-40 minutes, or until the quiche is set and the top is golden brown.

8. Remove from the oven and let it cool for a few minutes before slicing.

9. Garnish with chopped fresh parsley before serving.

10. Serve warm or at room temperature as a delicious breakfast, brunch, or light dinner option.

Nutritional Values (Approximate, per serving):

Calories: 250-300 kcal | Protein: 15-18 grams | Fat: 18-20 grams | Saturated Fat: 7-9 grams | Carbohydrates: 4-6 grams | Dietary Fiber: 1-2 grams | Sugars: 2-3 grams

Scrambled Eggs with Spinach:

Prep Time: 10 minutes   **Servings:** 2

Ingredients:

- 4 large eggs

- 1 cup fresh spinach leaves

- 2 tablespoons milk

- Salt and pepper, to taste

- 1 tablespoon olive oil or butter

Instructions:

1. In a bowl, beat the eggs with milk, salt, and pepper until well combined.

2. Heat olive oil or butter in a skillet over medium heat.

3. Add the spinach leaves to the skillet and cook until wilted.

4. Pour the beaten eggs into the skillet with the spinach.

5. Cook, stirring occasionally, until the eggs are scrambled and cooked to your desired consistency.

6. Serve hot as a nutritious breakfast option.

Nutritional Values (Approximate, per serving):

Calories: 150-200 kcal | Protein: 12-15 grams | Fat: 10-12 grams | Saturated Fat: 3-5 grams | Carbohydrates: 2-4 grams | Dietary Fiber: 1-2 grams | Sugars: 1-2 grams

Omelet Wraps:

Prep Time: 10 minutes　　　　　　**Servings**: 2

Ingredients:

- 4 large eggs

- 1/4 cup milk

- Salt and pepper, to taste

- 1 tablespoon olive oil or butter

- Fillings of your choice (e.g., diced bell peppers, onions, tomatoes, cheese, ham)

Instructions:

1. In a bowl, whisk together the eggs, milk, salt, and pepper until well combined.

2. Heat olive oil or butter in a non-stick skillet over medium heat.

3. Pour half of the egg mixture into the skillet, swirling to coat the bottom evenly.

4. Cook until the edges start to set, then add your desired fillings to one half of the omelet.

5. Carefully fold the other half of the omelet over the fillings to create a half-moon shape.

6. Cook for another 1-2 minutes until the omelet is cooked through and the fillings are heated.

7. Repeat with the remaining egg mixture to make the second omelet.

8. Serve hot as a versatile and satisfying meal.

Nutritional Values (Approximate, per serving):

Calories: 200-250 kcal | Protein: 12-15 grams | Fat: 14-16 grams | Saturated Fat: 5-7 grams | Carbohydrates: 2-4 grams | Dietary Fiber: 0 grams | Sugars: 1-2 grams

Light Omelet with Chicken and Spinach:

Prep Time: 15 minutes   **Servings**: 2

Ingredients:

- 4 large eggs

- 1/4 cup milk

- Salt and pepper, to taste

- 1 tablespoon olive oil

- 1 cup cooked chicken breast, diced

- 1 cup fresh spinach leaves

- 1/4 cup shredded mozzarella cheese (optional)

Instructions:

1. In a bowl, whisk together the eggs, milk, salt, and pepper until well combined.

2. Heat olive oil in a non-stick skillet over medium heat.

3. Add the diced chicken breast to the skillet and cook until heated through.

4. Add the fresh spinach leaves to the skillet and cook until wilted.

5. Pour the egg mixture over the chicken and spinach in the skillet.

6. Cook until the edges start to set, then sprinkle shredded mozzarella cheese over one half of the omelet, if desired.

7. Carefully fold the other half of the omelet over the cheese to create a half-moon shape.

8. Cook for another 1-2 minutes until the omelet is cooked through and the cheese is melted.

9. Serve hot as a light and protein-rich meal option.

Nutritional Values (Approximate, per serving):

Calories: 250-300 kcal | Protein: 25-30 grams | Fat: 15-18 grams | Saturated Fat: 4-6 grams | Carbohydrates: 2-4 grams | Dietary Fiber: 1-2 grams | Sugars: 1-2 grams

Roasted Sweet Potato and Bell Pepper Frittata:

Prep Time: 15 minutes   **Servings**: 4

Ingredients:

- 6 large eggs

- 1 medium sweet potato, peeled and diced

- 1 bell pepper, diced

- 1/2 onion, diced

- 1 tablespoon olive oil

- Salt and pepper, to taste

- 1/4 cup shredded cheddar cheese (optional)

- Fresh parsley, chopped, for garnish

Instructions:

1. Preheat your oven to 400°F (200°C).

2. In a large oven-safe skillet, heat olive oil over medium heat.

3. Add diced sweet potato, bell pepper, and onion to the skillet. Cook until vegetables are tender, about 8-10 minutes.

4. In a bowl, whisk together eggs, salt, and pepper.

5. Pour the egg mixture over the cooked vegetables in the skillet.

6. Sprinkle shredded cheddar cheese over the top, if using.

7. Transfer the skillet to the preheated oven and bake for 12-15 minutes, or until the frittata is set and golden brown.

8. Remove from the oven and let it cool for a few minutes before slicing.

9. Garnish with chopped fresh parsley before serving.

10. Serve warm or at room temperature as a hearty breakfast or brunch option.

Nutritional Values (Approximate, per serving):

Calories: 200-250 kcal | Protein: 10-12 grams | Fat: 12-15 grams | Saturated Fat: 3-5 grams | Carbohydrates: 10-12 grams | Dietary Fiber: 2-4 grams | Sugars: 3-4 grams

Cheese and Herb Scones:

Prep Time: 20 minutes   **Servings**: 6

Ingredients:

- 2 cups all-purpose flour

- 1 tablespoon baking powder

- 1/2 teaspoon salt

- 1/4 cup unsalted butter, cold and cubed

- 1 cup shredded cheddar cheese

- 1 tablespoon fresh parsley, finely chopped

- 1/2 cup milk

Instructions:

1. Preheat your oven to 400°F (200°C). Line a baking sheet with parchment paper.

2. In a large bowl, whisk together flour, baking powder, and salt.

3. Add cold cubed butter to the flour mixture. Using your fingers or a pastry cutter, rub the butter into the flour until the mixture resembles coarse crumbs.

4. Stir in shredded cheddar cheese and chopped parsley.

5. Gradually add milk to the mixture, stirring until a dough forms.

6. Turn the dough out onto a lightly floured surface and gently knead a few times until it comes together.

7. Pat the dough into a circle about 1-inch thick. Use a sharp knife to cut the circle into 6 equal wedges.

8. Place the scones onto the prepared baking sheet.

9. Bake for 15-18 minutes, or until the scones are golden brown and cooked through.

10. Remove from the oven and let them cool slightly before serving.

11. Serve warm with butter or your favorite spread.

Nutritional Values (Approximate, per serving):

Calories: 250-300 kcal | Protein: 8-10 grams | Fat: 12-15 grams | Saturated Fat: 7-9 grams | Carbohydrates: 25-30 grams | Dietary Fiber: 1-2 grams | Sugars: 1-2 grams

Chocolate Scones:

Prep Time: 15 minutes   **Servings**: 6

Ingredients:

- 2 cups all-purpose flour

- 1/3 cup cocoa powder

- 1/3 cup granulated sugar

- 1 tablespoon baking powder

- 1/2 teaspoon salt

- 1/2 cup unsalted butter, cold and cubed

- 1/2 cup milk

- 1 teaspoon vanilla extract

- 1/2 cup chocolate chips

Instructions:

1. Preheat your oven to 400°F (200°C). Line a baking sheet with parchment paper.

2. In a large bowl, whisk together flour, cocoa powder, sugar, baking powder, and salt.

3. Add cold cubed butter to the flour mixture. Using your fingers or a pastry cutter, rub the butter into the flour until the mixture resembles coarse crumbs.

4. Stir in chocolate chips.

5. In a separate bowl, whisk together milk and vanilla extract.

6. Gradually add the milk mixture to the dry ingredients, stirring until a dough forms.

7. Turn the dough out onto a lightly floured surface and gently knead a few times until it comes together.

8. Pat the dough into a circle about 1-inch thick. Use a sharp knife to cut the circle into 6 equal wedges.

9. Place the scones onto the prepared baking sheet.

10. Bake for 15-18 minutes, or until the scones are set and cooked through.

11. Remove from the oven and let them cool slightly before serving.

12. Serve warm or at room temperature with a dusting of cocoa powder or powdered sugar, if desired.

Nutritional Values (Approximate, per serving):

Calories: 300-350 kcal | Protein: 5-7 grams | Fat: 15-18 grams | Saturated Fat: 9-11 grams | Carbohydrates: 40-45 grams | Dietary Fiber: 2-4 grams | Sugars: 15-20 grams

Blueberry Pancakes:

Prep Time: 10 minutes   **Cook Time**: 10 minutes   **Servings**: 4

Ingredients:

- 1 cup all-purpose flour

- 2 tablespoons granulated sugar

- 1 tablespoon baking powder

- 1/4 teaspoon salt

- 1 egg

- 3/4 cup milk

- 2 tablespoons unsalted butter, melted

- 1 teaspoon vanilla extract

- 1 cup fresh or frozen blueberries

Instructions:

1. In a large bowl, whisk together flour, sugar, baking powder, and salt.

2. In another bowl, whisk together egg, milk, melted butter, and vanilla extract.

3. Pour the wet ingredients into the dry ingredients and stir until just combined. Do not overmix; a few lumps are okay.

4. Gently fold in the blueberries.

5. Heat a lightly greased skillet or griddle over medium heat.

6. Pour about 1/4 cup of batter onto the skillet for each pancake.

7. Cook until bubbles form on the surface of the pancakes and the edges look set, about 2-3 minutes.

8. Flip the pancakes and cook for another 1-2 minutes, or until golden brown and cooked through.

9. Repeat with the remaining batter.

10. Serve warm with maple syrup or your favorite toppings.

Nutritional Values (Approximate, per serving):

Calories: 200-250 kcal | Protein: 5-7 grams | Fat: 6-8 grams | Saturated Fat: 3-4 grams | Carbohydrates: 30-35 grams | Dietary Fiber: 2-3 grams | Sugars: 8-10 grams

Banana Pancakes:

Prep Time: 10 minutes   **Cook Time:** 10 minutes   **Servings:** 4

Ingredients:

- 2 ripe bananas

- 2 large eggs

- 1/2 cup oat flour or finely ground oats

- 1 teaspoon baking powder

- 1/2 teaspoon ground cinnamon (optional)

- 1/4 teaspoon salt

- Butter or oil for cooking

Instructions:

1. In a mixing bowl, mash the ripe bananas until smooth.

2. Add the eggs to the mashed bananas and whisk until well combined.

3. Stir in oat flour, baking powder, ground cinnamon (if using), and salt until a smooth batter forms.

4. Heat a non-stick skillet or griddle over medium heat and lightly grease with butter or oil.

5. Pour about 1/4 cup of batter onto the skillet for each pancake.

6. Cook until bubbles form on the surface of the pancakes and the edges look set, about 2-3 minutes.

7. Flip the pancakes and cook for another 1-2 minutes, or until golden brown and cooked through.

8. Repeat with the remaining batter.

9. Serve warm with sliced bananas, maple syrup, or your favorite toppings.

Nutritional Values (Approximate, per serving):

Calories: 150-200 kcal | Protein: 6-8 grams | Fat: 5-7 grams | Saturated Fat: 1-2 grams | Carbohydrates: 20-25 grams | Dietary Fiber: 2-4 grams | Sugars: 8-10 grams

Rice Cake with Almond Butter:

Prep Time: 5 minutes   **Servings:** 1

Ingredients:

- 1 rice cake

- 1-2 tablespoons almond butter

- Sliced banana or berries (optional)

- Honey or maple syrup (optional)

- Chia seeds or shredded coconut (optional)

Instructions:

1. Spread almond butter evenly over the rice cake.

2. Top with sliced banana or berries, if desired.

3. Drizzle with honey or maple syrup for added sweetness, if desired.

4. Sprinkle with chia seeds or shredded coconut for extra texture, if desired.

5. Serve as a quick and satisfying snack or breakfast option.

Nutritional Values (Approximate, per serving): Calories: 150-200 kcal | Protein: 4-6 grams | Fat: 8-10 grams | Saturated Fat: 1-2 grams | Carbohydrates: 15-20 grams | Dietary Fiber: 2-3 grams | Sugars: 3-5 grams

Smoothie with Tofu:

Prep Time: 5 minutes   **Servings**: 1

Ingredients:

- 1/2 cup silken tofu

- 1/2 cup frozen mixed berries

- 1 ripe banana

- 1/2 cup spinach leaves

- 1/2 cup unsweetened almond milk (or any milk of your choice)

- 1 tablespoon honey or maple syrup (optional)

- Ice cubes (optional)

Instructions:

1. In a blender, combine silken tofu, frozen mixed berries, banana, spinach leaves, almond milk, and honey or maple syrup (if using).

2. Blend until smooth and creamy. If the smoothie is too thick, you can add more almond milk or water to reach your desired consistency.

3. If desired, add ice cubes and blend again until smooth.

4. Pour the smoothie into a glass and serve immediately as a nutritious and protein-packed breakfast or snack option.

Nutritional Values (Approximate, per serving):

Calories: 250-300 kcal | Protein: 12-15 grams | Fat: 5-7 grams | Saturated Fat: 1-2 grams | Carbohydrates: 35-40 grams | Dietary Fiber: 6-8 grams | Sugars: 20-25 grams

Egg Muffins:

Prep Time: 10 minutes   **Cook Time**: 20 minutes   **Servings**: 6

Ingredients:

- 6 large eggs
- 1/4 cup milk
- Salt and pepper, to taste
- Fillings of your choice (e.g., diced vegetables, cooked bacon or sausage, shredded cheese)
- Cooking spray or oil for greasing

Instructions:

1. Preheat your oven to 350°F (175°C). Grease a 6-cup muffin tin with cooking spray or oil.
2. In a bowl, whisk together eggs, milk, salt, and pepper until well combined.
3. Divide your choice of fillings evenly among the muffin cups.
4. Pour the egg mixture over the fillings in each muffin cup, filling about 3/4 full.
5. Gently stir the fillings and egg mixture in each muffin cup to distribute evenly.
6. Bake in the preheated oven for 20-25 minutes, or until the egg muffins are set and golden brown on top.
7. Remove from the oven and let them cool for a few minutes before removing from the muffin tin.
8. Serve warm or at room temperature as a convenient and protein-rich breakfast option.

Nutritional Values (Approximate, per serving):

Calories: 100-150 kcal | Protein: 8-10 grams | Fat: 6-8 grams | Saturated Fat: 2-3 grams | Carbohydrates: 2-4 grams | Dietary Fiber: 0 grams | Sugars: 1-2 grams

Chia Seed Pudding:

Prep Time: 5 minutes   **Refrigeration Time**: 2 hours (or overnight)   **Servings**: 2

Ingredients:

- 1/4 cup chia seeds
- 1 cup unsweetened almond milk (or any milk of your choice)
- 1 tablespoon honey or maple syrup (optional)
- 1/2 teaspoon vanilla extract
- Fresh fruits, nuts, or seeds for topping (optional)

Instructions:

1. In a bowl or jar, mix together chia seeds, almond milk, honey or maple syrup (if using), and vanilla extract until well combined.
2. Cover the bowl or jar and refrigerate for at least 2 hours or overnight, allowing the chia seeds to absorb the liquid and thicken.
3. Stir the chia seed mixture before serving to redistribute any settled seeds.
4. Serve the chia seed pudding cold, topped with your favorite fruits, nuts, or seeds for added flavor and texture.
5. Enjoy as a delicious and nutrient-rich breakfast or snack option.

Nutritional Values (Approximate, per serving): Calories: 150-200 kcal | Protein: 4-6 grams | Fat: 8-10 grams | Saturated Fat: 1-2 grams | Carbohydrates: 15-20 grams | Dietary Fiber: 8-10 grams | Sugars: 5-8 grams

Quinoa Breakfast Bowl:

Prep Time: 10 minutes   **Cook Time**: 15 minutes   **Servings**: 2

Ingredients:

- 1/2 cup quinoa, rinsed

- 1 cup water or vegetable broth

- 1/2 teaspoon ground cinnamon

- 1 tablespoon honey or maple syrup (optional)

- 1/2 cup Greek yogurt or dairy-free yogurt

- Fresh fruits, nuts, seeds, or granola for topping

Instructions:

1. In a small saucepan, combine quinoa, water or vegetable broth, ground cinnamon, and honey or maple syrup (if using).

2. Bring the mixture to a boil, then reduce the heat to low and simmer, covered, for 15 minutes, or until the quinoa is cooked and the liquid is absorbed.

3. Remove the saucepan from the heat and let it sit, covered, for 5 minutes.

4. Fluff the quinoa with a fork and divide it into serving bowls.

5. Top the quinoa with Greek yogurt or dairy-free yogurt.

6. Add your choice of fresh fruits, nuts, seeds, or granola as toppings.

7. Serve the quinoa breakfast bowl warm or chilled, as a nutritious and satisfying breakfast option.

Nutritional Values (Approximate, per serving):

Calories: 250-300 kcal | Protein: 10-12 grams | Fat: 4-6 grams | Saturated Fat: 1-2 grams | Carbohydrates: 40-45 grams | Dietary Fiber: 5-8 grams | Sugars: 8-10 grams

CHAPTER FIVE:

LUNCH

Caprese Quinoa Salad:

Prep Time: 15 minutes   **Cook Time:** 15 minutes   **Servings**: 4

Ingredients:

- 1 cup quinoa, rinsed

- 2 cups water or vegetable broth

- 1 cup cherry tomatoes, halved

- 1 cup fresh mozzarella balls, halved

- 1/4 cup fresh basil leaves, chopped

- 2 tablespoons extra virgin olive oil

- 1 tablespoon balsamic vinegar

- Salt and pepper, to taste

Instructions:

1. In a medium saucepan, combine quinoa and water or vegetable broth. Bring to a boil, then reduce heat to low, cover, and simmer for 15 minutes, or until quinoa is cooked and liquid is absorbed.

2. Fluff the cooked quinoa with a fork and let it cool to room temperature.

3. In a large bowl, combine cooked quinoa, halved cherry tomatoes, halved mozzarella balls, and chopped fresh basil.

4. Drizzle extra virgin olive oil and balsamic vinegar over the salad.

5. Season with salt and pepper to taste, and toss gently to combine.

6. Serve the Caprese quinoa salad as a refreshing side dish or light meal.

Nutritional Values (Approximate, per serving):

Calories: 250-300 kcal | Protein: 10-12 grams | Fat: 14-16 grams | Saturated Fat: 5-7 grams |
Carbohydrates: 20-25 grams | Dietary Fiber: 3-5 grams | Sugars: 2-3 grams

Rice Vegetable Soup:

Prep Time: 10 minutes   **Cook Time:** 30 minutes   **Servings:** 4

Ingredients:

- 1 tablespoon olive oil
- 1 onion, diced
- 2 cloves garlic, minced
- 2 carrots, diced
- 2 celery stalks, diced
- 1 bell pepper, diced
- 1 cup diced tomatoes (fresh or canned)
- 1/2 cup long-grain white rice
- 4 cups vegetable broth
- 1 teaspoon dried thyme
- Salt and pepper, to taste
- Fresh parsley, chopped, for garnish (optional)

Instructions:

1. In a large pot, heat olive oil over medium heat. Add diced onion and garlic, and sauté until softened and fragrant, about 5 minutes.

2. Add diced carrots, celery, and bell pepper to the pot, and cook for another 5 minutes, or until vegetables are slightly tender.

3. Stir in diced tomatoes, white rice, vegetable broth, and dried thyme. Bring to a boil.

4. Reduce heat to low, cover, and simmer for 20-25 minutes, or until the rice is cooked and the vegetables are tender.

5. Season with salt and pepper to taste, adjusting as needed.

6. Serve the rice vegetable soup hot, garnished with chopped fresh parsley if desired.

Nutritional Values (Approximate, per serving):

Calories: 200-250 kcal | Protein: 4-6 grams | Fat: 4-6 grams | Saturated Fat: 1 gram | Carbohydrates: 35-40 grams | Dietary Fiber: 4-6 grams | Sugars: 6-8 grams

Veggie Stir-Fry with Tofu:

Prep Time: 15 minutes   **Cook Time**: 15 minutes   **Servings**: 4

Ingredients:

- 14 oz (400g) firm tofu, drained and cubed

- 2 tablespoons soy sauce

- 2 tablespoons cornstarch

- 2 tablespoons vegetable oil

- 2 cloves garlic, minced

- 1 tablespoon ginger, minced

- 1 red bell pepper, sliced

- 1 yellow bell pepper, sliced

- 1 cup broccoli florets

- 1 cup snow peas

- 1 carrot, julienned

- 1/4 cup soy sauce (for stir-fry sauce)

- 2 tablespoons hoisin sauce (for stir-fry sauce)

- 1 tablespoon sesame oil (for stir-fry sauce)

- Cooked rice or noodles, for serving

Instructions:

1. In a bowl, toss the cubed tofu with 2 tablespoons of soy sauce and cornstarch until evenly coated.

2. Heat 1 tablespoon of vegetable oil in a large skillet or wok over medium-high heat. Add the tofu cubes and cook until golden brown on all sides, about 5-7 minutes. Remove the tofu from the skillet and set aside.

3. In the same skillet, add the remaining tablespoon of vegetable oil. Add minced garlic and ginger, and cook for about 1 minute until fragrant.

4. Add sliced bell peppers, broccoli florets, snow peas, and julienned carrot to the skillet. Stir-fry for 5-7 minutes until the vegetables are tender-crisp.

5. Return the cooked tofu to the skillet with the vegetables.

6. In a small bowl, whisk together 1/4 cup soy sauce, hoisin sauce, and sesame oil to make the stir-fry sauce.

7. Pour the stir-fry sauce over the tofu and vegetables in the skillet. Stir well to coat everything evenly.

8. Cook for another 2-3 minutes until the sauce thickens and coats the tofu and vegetables.

9. Serve the veggie stir-fry with tofu hot over cooked rice or noodles.

Nutritional Values (Approximate, per serving):

Calories: 250-300 kcal | Protein: 15-18 grams | Fat: 12-15 grams | Saturated Fat: 2-3 grams | Carbohydrates: 20-25 grams | Dietary Fiber: 4-6 grams | Sugars: 6-8 grams

Beef and Broccoli Stir-Fry:

Prep Time: 15 minutes   **Cook Time:** 15 minutes   **Servings:** 4

Ingredients:

- 1 lb (450g) flank steak, thinly sliced

- 3 cups broccoli florets

- 1 tablespoon vegetable oil

- 3 cloves garlic, minced

- 1 teaspoon ginger, minced

- 1/4 cup soy sauce

- 2 tablespoons oyster sauce

- 1 tablespoon hoisin sauce

- 1 tablespoon cornstarch

- 1/4 cup water

- Cooked rice, for serving

- Sesame seeds, for garnish (optional)

Instructions:

1. In a bowl, marinate the thinly sliced flank steak with soy sauce for about 10 minutes.

2. In a small bowl, mix together oyster sauce, hoisin sauce, cornstarch, and water to make the stir-fry sauce. Set aside.

3. Heat vegetable oil in a large skillet or wok over medium-high heat. Add minced garlic and ginger, and cook for about 1 minute until fragrant.

4. Add the marinated flank steak to the skillet and stir-fry for 2-3 minutes until browned. Remove the beef from the skillet and set aside.

5. In the same skillet, add broccoli florets and stir-fry for 3-4 minutes until tender-crisp.

6. Return the cooked beef to the skillet with the broccoli.

7. Pour the stir-fry sauce over the beef and broccoli in the skillet. Stir well to coat everything evenly.

8. Cook for another 2-3 minutes until the sauce thickens and coats the beef and broccoli.

9. Serve the beef and broccoli stir-fry hot over cooked rice, garnished with sesame seeds if desired.

Nutritional Values (Approximate, per serving):

Calories: 250-300 kcal | Protein: 25-30 grams | Fat: 10-12 grams | Saturated Fat: 3-4 grams | Carbohydrates: 15-20 grams | Dietary Fiber: 3-5 grams | Sugars: 3-5 grams

Baked Salmon with Lemon and Dill:

Prep Time: 5 minutes   **Cook Time**: 15 minutes   **Servings**: 4

Ingredients:

- 4 salmon fillets (about 6 oz each)
- Salt and pepper, to taste
- 2 tablespoons olive oil
- 2 tablespoons lemon juice
- 2 cloves garlic, minced
- 1 tablespoon fresh dill, chopped
- Lemon slices, for garnish

Instructions:

1. Preheat your oven to 400°F (200°C). Line a baking sheet with parchment paper.
2. Season salmon fillets with salt and pepper on both sides.
3. In a small bowl, whisk together olive oil, lemon juice, minced garlic, and chopped dill.
4. Place the seasoned salmon fillets on the prepared baking sheet.
5. Drizzle the lemon-dill mixture over the salmon fillets, making sure to coat them evenly.
6. Place a lemon slice on top of each salmon fillet for extra flavor.
7. Bake in the preheated oven for 12-15 minutes, or until the salmon is cooked through and flakes easily with a fork.
8. Remove from the oven and let it rest for a few minutes before serving.
9. Serve the baked salmon hot, garnished with additional fresh dill and lemon slices if desired.

Nutritional Values (Approximate, per serving):

Calories: 250-300 kcal | Protein: 25-30 grams | Fat: 15-18 grams | Saturated Fat: 2-3 grams | Carbohydrates: 2-3 grams | Dietary Fiber: 0 grams | Sugars: 0 grams

Mediterranean Quinoa Salad:

Prep Time: 15 minutes   **Cook Time**: 15 minutes   **Servings**: 4

Ingredients:

- 1 cup quinoa, rinsed

- 2 cups water or vegetable broth

- 1 cup cherry tomatoes, halved

- 1 cucumber, diced

- 1/2 cup Kalamata olives, pitted and halved

- 1/4 cup red onion, finely chopped

- 1/4 cup fresh parsley, chopped

- 1/4 cup fresh mint leaves, chopped

- 1/4 cup crumbled feta cheese

- 2 tablespoons extra virgin olive oil

- 2 tablespoons lemon juice

- 1 clove garlic, minced

- Salt and pepper, to taste

Instructions:

1. In a medium saucepan, combine quinoa and water or vegetable broth. Bring to a boil, then reduce heat to low, cover, and simmer for 15 minutes, or until quinoa is cooked and liquid is absorbed.

2. Fluff the cooked quinoa with a fork and let it cool to room temperature.

3. In a large bowl, combine cooked quinoa, halved cherry tomatoes, diced cucumber, halved Kalamata olives, finely chopped red onion, chopped parsley, chopped mint leaves, and crumbled feta cheese.

4. In a small bowl, whisk together extra virgin olive oil, lemon juice, minced garlic, salt, and pepper to make the dressing.

5. Pour the dressing over the quinoa salad and toss gently to coat everything evenly.

6. Taste and adjust seasoning if necessary.

7. Serve the Mediterranean quinoa salad chilled or at room temperature as a refreshing side dish or light meal.

Nutritional Values (Approximate, per serving):

Calories: 250-300 kcal | Protein: 8-10 grams | Fat: 10-12 grams | Saturated Fat: 2-3 grams | Carbohydrates: 35-40 grams | Dietary Fiber: 5-7 grams | Sugars: 3-5 grams

Turkey Lettuce Wraps:

Prep Time: 10 minutes   **Cook Time:** 10 minutes   **Servings:** 4

Ingredients:

- 1 lb (450g) ground turkey
- 2 cloves garlic, minced
- 1 tablespoon ginger, minced
- 1/4 cup soy sauce
- 2 tablespoons hoisin sauce
- 1 tablespoon rice vinegar
- 1 teaspoon sesame oil
- 1 teaspoon sriracha sauce (optional)
- 1 cup shredded carrots

- 1 cup sliced bell peppers

- 1/4 cup green onions, sliced

- 1/4 cup fresh cilantro, chopped

- 1 head butter lettuce or iceberg lettuce, leaves separated

Instructions:

1. In a large skillet, cook ground turkey over medium-high heat until browned and cooked through, breaking it apart with a spoon as it cooks.

2. Add minced garlic and ginger to the skillet with the cooked turkey, and cook for 1-2 minutes until fragrant.

3. Stir in soy sauce, hoisin sauce, rice vinegar, sesame oil, and sriracha sauce (if using), and cook for another 2-3 minutes until heated through.

4. Add shredded carrots, sliced bell peppers, sliced green onions, and chopped cilantro to the skillet with the turkey mixture. Stir well to combine.

5. Cook for another 2-3 minutes until the vegetables are slightly softened.

6. Remove from heat and let the mixture cool slightly.

7. To serve, spoon the turkey mixture onto lettuce leaves and wrap them up like tacos.

8. Serve the turkey lettuce wraps immediately, with additional sriracha sauce or hoisin sauce for dipping if desired.

Nutritional Values (Approximate, per serving):

Calories: 200-250 kcal | Protein: 20-25 grams | Fat: 8-10 grams | Saturated Fat: 2-3 grams | Carbohydrates: 15-20 grams | Dietary Fiber: 3-5 grams | Sugars: 5-7 grams

Chickpea Salad:

Prep Time: 10 minutes   **Servings**: 4

Ingredients:

- 2 cups cooked chickpeas (or 1 can, drained and rinsed)
- 1 cucumber, diced
- 1 bell pepper, diced
- 1/4 cup red onion, finely chopped
- 1/4 cup fresh parsley, chopped
- 2 tablespoons fresh lemon juice
- 2 tablespoons extra virgin olive oil
- 1 teaspoon ground cumin
- Salt and pepper, to taste

Instructions:

1. In a large bowl, combine cooked chickpeas, diced cucumber, diced bell pepper, finely chopped red onion, and chopped parsley.

2. In a small bowl, whisk together fresh lemon juice, extra virgin olive oil, ground cumin, salt, and pepper to make the dressing.

3. Pour the dressing over the chickpea salad and toss gently to coat everything evenly.

4. Taste and adjust seasoning if necessary.

5. Serve the chickpea salad chilled or at room temperature as a refreshing side dish or light meal.

Nutritional Values (Approximate, per serving):

Calories: 200-250 kcal | Protein: 8-10 grams | Fat: 8-10 grams | Saturated Fat: 1-2 grams | Carbohydrates: 25-30 grams | Dietary Fiber: 6-8 grams | Sugars: 5-7 grams

Salmon and Brown Rice Bowl:

Prep Time: 10 minutes   **Cook Time**: 20 minutes   **Servings**: 4

Ingredients:

- 4 salmon fillets (about 6 oz each)
- Salt and pepper, to taste
- 2 cups cooked brown rice
- 2 cups mixed vegetables (such as broccoli, carrots, and bell peppers), steamed
- 2 tablespoons soy sauce
- 1 tablespoon honey
- 1 tablespoon sesame oil
- 1 tablespoon rice vinegar
- Sesame seeds, for garnish
- Sliced green onions, for garnish

Instructions:

1. Preheat your oven to 400°F (200°C). Line a baking sheet with parchment paper.
2. Season salmon fillets with salt and pepper on both sides.
3. Place the seasoned salmon fillets on the prepared baking sheet.
4. In a small bowl, whisk together soy sauce, honey, sesame oil, and rice vinegar to make the glaze.
5. Brush the glaze over the salmon fillets.
6. Bake in the preheated oven for 12-15 minutes, or until the salmon is cooked through and flakes easily with a fork.
7. Divide cooked brown rice among serving bowls.
8. Top each bowl with steamed mixed vegetables and a baked salmon fillet.

9. Garnish with sesame seeds and sliced green onions.

10. Serve the salmon and brown rice bowls hot, drizzled with additional glaze if desired.

Nutritional Values (Approximate, per serving):

Calories: 350-400 kcal | Protein: 25-30 grams | Fat: 12-15 grams | Saturated Fat: 2-3 grams | Carbohydrates: 30-35 grams | Dietary Fiber: 4-6 grams | Sugars: 6-8 grams

Quinoa Stuffed Bell Peppers:

Prep Time: 15 minutes   **Cook Time**: 30 minutes   **Servings**: 4

Ingredients:

- 4 bell peppers (any color), halved and seeds removed

- 1 cup quinoa, rinsed

- 2 cups vegetable broth

- 1 tablespoon olive oil

- 1 onion, diced

- 2 cloves garlic, minced

- 1 zucchini, diced

- 1 carrot, diced

- 1 cup diced tomatoes (fresh or canned)

- 1 teaspoon dried oregano

- 1 teaspoon dried basil

- Salt and pepper, to taste

- 1/4 cup grated Parmesan cheese (optional)

- Fresh parsley, chopped, for garnish

Instructions:

1. Preheat your oven to 375°F (190°C).

2. In a medium saucepan, combine quinoa and vegetable broth. Bring to a boil, then reduce heat to low, cover, and simmer for 15-20 minutes, or until quinoa is cooked and liquid is absorbed.

3. Heat olive oil in a large skillet over medium heat. Add diced onion and minced garlic, and cook until softened and fragrant, about 5 minutes.

4. Add diced zucchini and carrot to the skillet, and cook for another 5 minutes until vegetables are tender.

5. Stir in diced tomatoes, dried oregano, and dried basil. Season with salt and pepper to taste.

6. Add cooked quinoa to the skillet with the vegetable mixture. Stir well to combine.

7. Stuff each halved bell pepper with the quinoa and vegetable mixture.

8. Place stuffed bell peppers in a baking dish. Cover with aluminum foil and bake in the preheated oven for 20-25 minutes, or until the peppers are tender.

9. If desired, sprinkle grated Parmesan cheese over the stuffed peppers during the last 5 minutes of baking.

10. Remove from the oven and let cool slightly before serving.

11. Garnish with chopped fresh parsley before serving.

Nutritional Values (Approximate, per serving):

Calories: 250-300 kcal | Protein: 8-10 grams | Fat: 8-10 grams | Saturated Fat: 1-2 grams | Carbohydrates: 35-40 grams | Dietary Fiber: 6-8 grams | Sugars: 5-7 grams

Eggplant and Tomato Salad:

Prep Time: 15 minutes   **Cook Time**: 15 minutes   **Servings**: 4

Ingredients:

- 1 large eggplant, diced

- 2 tomatoes, diced

- 1/4 cup red onion, finely chopped

- 2 tablespoons extra virgin olive oil

- 1 tablespoon balsamic vinegar

- 2 cloves garlic, minced

- 1/4 cup fresh basil leaves, chopped

- Salt and pepper, to taste

Instructions:

1. Preheat a grill or grill pan over medium-high heat.

2. In a large bowl, toss diced eggplant with 1 tablespoon of olive oil until evenly coated.

3. Grill the diced eggplant for 5-7 minutes per side, or until tender and lightly charred. Remove from heat and let cool slightly.

4. In a separate bowl, combine diced tomatoes, finely chopped red onion, minced garlic, and chopped fresh basil.

5. Add grilled eggplant to the bowl with the tomato mixture.

6. Drizzle remaining tablespoon of olive oil and balsamic vinegar over the salad. Toss gently to combine.

7. Season with salt and pepper to taste.

8. Serve the eggplant and tomato salad chilled or at room temperature as a flavorful side dish or appetizer.

Nutritional Values (Approximate, per serving):

Calories: 150-200 kcal | Protein: 2-3 grams | Fat: 10-12 grams | Saturated Fat: 1-2 grams | Carbohydrates: 15-20 grams | Dietary Fiber: 6-8 grams | Sugars: 8-10 grams

Shrimp Stir-Fry:

Prep Time: 15 minutes   **Cook Time**: 10 minutes   **Servings**: 4

Ingredients:

- 1 lb (450g) shrimp, peeled and deveined
- 2 tablespoons soy sauce
- 1 tablespoon oyster sauce
- 1 tablespoon hoisin sauce
- 1 tablespoon sesame oil
- 2 tablespoons vegetable oil
- 3 cloves garlic, minced
- 1 tablespoon ginger, minced
- 1 bell pepper, thinly sliced
- 1 cup broccoli florets
- 1 carrot, julienned
- 1/2 cup snap peas
- Cooked rice or noodles, for serving
- Sesame seeds, for garnish
- Sliced green onions, for garnish

Instructions:

1. In a bowl, marinate the shrimp with soy sauce, oyster sauce, and hoisin sauce for about 10 minutes.

2. Heat sesame oil and vegetable oil in a large skillet or wok over medium-high heat.

3. Add minced garlic and ginger to the skillet and cook for about 1 minute until fragrant.

4. Add sliced bell pepper, broccoli florets, julienned carrot, and snap peas to the skillet. Stir-fry for 3-4 minutes until vegetables are tender-crisp.

5. Add marinated shrimp to the skillet and stir-fry for another 2-3 minutes until shrimp are pink and cooked through.

6. Serve the shrimp stir-fry hot over cooked rice or noodles.

7. Garnish with sesame seeds and sliced green onions before serving.

Nutritional Values (Approximate, per serving):

Calories: 200-250 kcal | Protein: 20-25 grams | Fat: 10-12 grams | Saturated Fat: 2-3 grams | Carbohydrates: 10-15 grams | Dietary Fiber: 2-3 grams | Sugars: 3-5 grams

Tuna Quinoa Salad:

Prep Time: 15 minutes   **Cook Time**: 15 minutes   **Servings**: 4

Ingredients:

- 1 cup quinoa, rinsed
- 2 cups water or vegetable broth
- 2 cans (5 oz each) tuna, drained
- 1 cucumber, diced
- 1 bell pepper, diced
- 1/4 cup red onion, finely chopped
- 1/4 cup Kalamata olives, pitted and halved
- 1/4 cup feta cheese, crumbled
- 2 tablespoons extra virgin olive oil
- 2 tablespoons lemon juice
- 1 teaspoon dried oregano
- Salt and pepper, to taste

Instructions:

1. In a medium saucepan, combine quinoa and water or vegetable broth. Bring to a boil, then reduce heat to low, cover, and simmer for 15 minutes, or until quinoa is cooked and liquid is absorbed.

2. Fluff the cooked quinoa with a fork and let it cool to room temperature.

3. In a large bowl, combine cooked quinoa, drained tuna, diced cucumber, diced bell pepper, finely chopped red onion, halved Kalamata olives, and crumbled feta cheese.

4. In a small bowl, whisk together extra virgin olive oil, lemon juice, dried oregano, salt, and pepper to make the dressing.

5. Pour the dressing over the tuna quinoa salad and toss gently to coat everything evenly.

6. Taste and adjust seasoning if necessary.

7. Serve the tuna quinoa salad chilled or at room temperature as a satisfying and nutritious meal.

Nutritional Values (Approximate, per serving):

Calories: 300-350 kcal | Protein: 20-25 grams | Fat: 12-15 grams | Saturated Fat: 3-4 grams | Carbohydrates: 25-30 grams | Dietary Fiber: 4-6 grams | Sugars: 3-5 grams

Chicken Salad Lettuce Wraps:

Prep Time: 15 minutes   **Cook Time**: 20 minutes   **Servings**: 4

Ingredients:

- 2 chicken breasts, cooked and shredded

- 1/2 cup Greek yogurt

- 2 tablespoons mayonnaise

- 1 tablespoon Dijon mustard

- 1 stalk celery, finely diced

- 1/4 cup red onion, finely chopped

- 1/4 cup grapes, halved

- 1/4 cup sliced almonds

- Salt and pepper, to taste

- 8 large lettuce leaves (such as iceberg or romaine)

Instructions:

1. In a large bowl, combine shredded chicken, Greek yogurt, mayonnaise, and Dijon mustard. Mix well until the chicken is coated evenly.

2. Add finely diced celery, finely chopped red onion, halved grapes, and sliced almonds to the chicken mixture.

3. Season with salt and pepper to taste, and stir until all ingredients are well combined.

4. Spoon the chicken salad mixture onto each lettuce leaf.

5. Wrap the lettuce leaves around the chicken salad mixture to form lettuce wraps.

6. Serve the chicken salad lettuce wraps immediately as a light and refreshing meal or appetizer.

Nutritional Values (Approximate, per serving):

Calories: 200-250 kcal | Protein: 20-25 grams | Fat: 8-10 grams | Saturated Fat: 1-2 grams | Carbohydrates: 10-15 grams | Dietary Fiber: 3-5 grams | Sugars: 5-7 grams

CHAPTER SIX:

DINNER

Grilled Chicken with Roasted Vegetables:

Prep Time: 15 minutes   **Cook Time**: 25 minutes   **Servings**: 4

Ingredients:

- 4 boneless, skinless chicken breasts

- 2 tablespoons olive oil

- 1 tablespoon balsamic vinegar

- 2 cloves garlic, minced

- 1 teaspoon dried Italian herbs (such as basil, oregano, and thyme)

- Salt and pepper, to taste

- 2 bell peppers, sliced

- 1 zucchini, sliced

- 1 yellow squash, sliced

- 1 red onion, sliced

- 1 cup cherry tomatoes

- Fresh parsley, chopped, for garnish

Instructions:

1. Preheat your grill to medium-high heat.

2. In a small bowl, whisk together olive oil, balsamic vinegar, minced garlic, dried Italian herbs, salt, and pepper to make the marinade.

3. Place chicken breasts in a shallow dish and pour the marinade over them. Allow to marinate for at least 15 minutes.

4. Meanwhile, preheat your oven to 400°F (200°C).

5. Arrange sliced bell peppers, zucchini, yellow squash, red onion, and cherry tomatoes on a baking sheet.

6. Drizzle with olive oil and season with salt and pepper. Toss to coat evenly.

7. Roast in the preheated oven for 20-25 minutes, or until vegetables are tender and slightly caramelized.

8. While vegetables are roasting, grill the marinated chicken breasts for 6-8 minutes per side, or until cooked through and no longer pink in the center.

9. Serve grilled chicken alongside roasted vegetables.

10. Garnish with chopped fresh parsley before serving.

Nutritional Values (Approximate, per serving):

Calories: 300-350 kcal | Protein: 30-35 grams | Fat: 10-12 grams | Saturated Fat: 2-3 grams | Carbohydrates: 20-25 grams | Dietary Fiber: 6-8 grams | Sugars: 8-10 grams

Turkey Meatballs with Zucchini Noodles:

Prep Time: 20 minutes   **Cook Time**: 20 minutes   **Servings**: 4

Ingredients:

- 1 lb (450g) lean ground turkey

- 1/4 cup breadcrumbs (gluten-free if desired)

- 1 egg

- 2 cloves garlic, minced

- 2 tablespoons fresh parsley, chopped

- 1 teaspoon dried oregano

- Salt and pepper, to taste

- 2 tablespoons olive oil

- 4 medium zucchini, spiralized into noodles

- 1 cup marinara sauce

- Grated Parmesan cheese, for serving (optional)

- Fresh basil leaves, torn, for garnish

Instructions:

1. In a large bowl, combine ground turkey, breadcrumbs, egg, minced garlic, chopped fresh parsley, dried oregano, salt, and pepper. Mix until well combined.

2. Shape the turkey mixture into meatballs, about 1 inch in diameter.

3. Heat olive oil in a large skillet over medium heat. Add the turkey meatballs to the skillet and cook for 8-10 minutes, turning occasionally, until browned and cooked through.

4. Remove the cooked meatballs from the skillet and set aside.

5. In the same skillet, add spiralized zucchini noodles and marinara sauce. Cook for 5-6 minutes, stirring occasionally, until the zucchini noodles are tender.

6. Return the cooked turkey meatballs to the skillet with the zucchini noodles and marinara sauce. Toss gently to combine and heat through.

7. Serve the turkey meatballs and zucchini noodles hot, garnished with grated Parmesan cheese and torn fresh basil leaves.

Nutritional Values (Approximate, per serving):

Calories: 250-300 kcal | Protein: 25-30 grams | Fat: 10-12 grams | Saturated Fat: 2-3 grams | Carbohydrates: 15-20 grams | Dietary Fiber: 4-6 grams | Sugars: 5-7 grams

Stir-Fried Tofu with Bok Choy:

Prep Time: 15 minutes   **Cook Time:** 10 minutes   **Servings:** 4

Ingredients:

- 1 block firm tofu, drained and cubed
- 2 tablespoons soy sauce
- 1 tablespoon hoisin sauce
- 1 tablespoon rice vinegar
- 1 tablespoon sesame oil
- 2 cloves garlic, minced
- 1 tablespoon ginger, minced
- 1 bunch baby bok choy, chopped
- 1 bell pepper, thinly sliced
- 2 green onions, sliced
- Cooked rice, for serving
- Sesame seeds, for garnish

Instructions:

1. In a small bowl, whisk together soy sauce, hoisin sauce, rice vinegar, and sesame oil to make the sauce.

2. Heat some oil in a large skillet or wok over medium-high heat.

3. Add cubed tofu to the skillet and cook until golden brown on all sides, about 5-6 minutes. Remove tofu from the skillet and set aside.

4. In the same skillet, add minced garlic and ginger. Stir-fry for about 1 minute until fragrant.

5. Add chopped bok choy and thinly sliced bell pepper to the skillet. Stir-fry for 2-3 minutes until vegetables are tender-crisp.

6. Return the cooked tofu to the skillet and pour the sauce over the tofu and vegetables.

7. Stir well to coat everything evenly and cook for another 1-2 minutes until heated through.

8. Serve the stir-fried tofu and bok choy hot over cooked rice.

9. Garnish with sliced green onions and sesame seeds before serving.

Nutritional Values (Approximate, per serving):

Calories: 200-250 kcal | Protein: 15-20 grams | Fat: 10-12 grams | Saturated Fat: 2-3 grams | Carbohydrates: 15-20 grams | Dietary Fiber: 4-6 grams | Sugars: 4-6 grams

Salmon and Asparagus Foil Packets:

Prep Time: 10 minutes **Cook Time:** 20 minutes **Servings:** 4

Ingredients:

- 4 salmon fillets (about 6 oz each)
- 1 lb (450g) asparagus, trimmed
- 2 tablespoons olive oil
- 2 cloves garlic, minced
- 1 lemon, thinly sliced
- Salt and pepper, to taste
- Fresh dill, for garnish

Instructions:

1. Preheat your oven to 400°F (200°C).
2. Tear off four large sheets of aluminum foil.
3. Place a salmon fillet in the center of each foil sheet.
4. Divide trimmed asparagus evenly among the foil packets, arranging them around the salmon fillets.
5. Drizzle olive oil over each salmon fillet and asparagus. Season with minced garlic, salt, and pepper.
6. Place two lemon slices on top of each salmon fillet.
7. Fold up the edges of the foil to create packets, sealing them tightly.
8. Place the foil packets on a baking sheet and bake in the preheated oven for 15-20 minutes, or until salmon is cooked through and flakes easily with a fork.
9. Carefully open the foil packets and transfer salmon and asparagus to serving plates.
10. Garnish with fresh dill before serving.

Nutritional Values (Approximate, per serving):

Calories: 300-350 kcal | Protein: 25-30 grams | Fat: 15-20 grams | Saturated Fat: 2-3 grams | Carbohydrates: 10-15 grams | Dietary Fiber: 5-7 grams | Sugars: 3-5 grams

Pork Tenderloin with Quinoa Pilaf:

Prep Time: 15 minutes   **Cook Time**: 25 minutes   **Servings**: 4

Ingredients:

- 1 lb (450g) pork tenderloin
- 2 tablespoons olive oil
- 2 cloves garlic, minced
- 1 teaspoon dried thyme
- 1 teaspoon dried rosemary
- Salt and pepper, to taste
- 1 cup quinoa, rinsed
- 2 cups chicken or vegetable broth
- 1/4 cup sliced almonds
- 1/4 cup dried cranberries
- Fresh parsley, chopped, for garnish

Instructions:

1. Preheat your oven to 400°F (200°C).

2. Rub pork tenderloin with olive oil, minced garlic, dried thyme, dried rosemary, salt, and pepper.

3. Place the seasoned pork tenderloin on a baking sheet lined with parchment paper.

4. Roast in the preheated oven for 20-25 minutes, or until pork reaches an internal temperature of 145°F (63°C).

5. While the pork is cooking, rinse quinoa under cold water and drain.

6. In a medium saucepan, bring chicken or vegetable broth to a boil. Stir in rinsed quinoa.

7. Reduce heat to low, cover, and simmer for 15 minutes, or until quinoa is cooked and liquid is absorbed.

8. Fluff the cooked quinoa with a fork and stir in sliced almonds and dried cranberries.

9. Slice the roasted pork tenderloin and serve it with quinoa pilaf.

10. Garnish with chopped fresh parsley before serving.

Nutritional Values (Approximate, per serving):

Calories: 300-350 kcal | Protein: 25-30 grams | Fat: 10-12 grams | Saturated Fat: 2-3 grams | Carbohydrates: 25-30 grams | Dietary Fiber: 4-6 grams | Sugars: 3-5 grams

Eggplant Parmesan:

Prep Time: 20 minutes   **Cook Time**: 40 minutes   **Servings**: 4

Ingredients:

- 2 large eggplants, sliced into rounds

- 2 eggs, beaten

- 1 cup breadcrumbs (gluten-free if desired)

- 1 cup marinara sauce

- 1 cup shredded mozzarella cheese

- 1/4 cup grated Parmesan cheese

- Fresh basil leaves, torn, for garnish

Instructions:

1. Preheat your oven to 375°F (190°C). Line a baking sheet with parchment paper.

2. Dip eggplant slices into beaten eggs, then coat with breadcrumbs.

3. Place coated eggplant slices on the prepared baking sheet.

4. Bake in the preheated oven for 20-25 minutes, or until eggplant is tender and golden brown.

5. Remove baked eggplant slices from the oven and reduce the oven temperature to 350°F (175°C).

6. In a baking dish, spread a thin layer of marinara sauce.

7. Arrange half of the baked eggplant slices in the baking dish.

8. Top eggplant slices with more marinara sauce, shredded mozzarella cheese, and grated Parmesan cheese.

9. Repeat layers with the remaining baked eggplant slices, marinara sauce, and cheeses.

10. Bake in the preheated oven for 20 minutes, or until cheese is melted and bubbly.

11. Garnish with torn fresh basil leaves before serving.

Nutritional Values (Approximate, per serving):

Calories: 250-300 kcal | Protein: 12-15 grams | Fat: 10-12 grams | Saturated Fat: 3-4 grams | Carbohydrates: 30-35 grams | Dietary Fiber: 6-8 grams | Sugars: 10-12 grams

Shrimp and Vegetable Skewers:

Prep Time: 20 minutes   **Cook Time**: 10 minutes   **Servings**: 4

Ingredients:

- 1 lb (450g) large shrimp, peeled and deveined
- 2 bell peppers, cut into chunks
- 1 red onion, cut into chunks
- 1 zucchini, sliced
- 1 lemon, sliced
- 2 tablespoons olive oil
- 2 cloves garlic, minced
- 1 teaspoon smoked paprika
- 1 teaspoon dried oregano
- Salt and pepper, to taste
- Wooden skewers, soaked in water for 30 minutes

Instructions:

1. Preheat your grill or grill pan to medium-high heat.

2. In a small bowl, whisk together olive oil, minced garlic, smoked paprika, dried oregano, salt, and pepper to make the marinade.

3. Thread shrimp, bell pepper chunks, red onion chunks, zucchini slices, and lemon slices onto the soaked wooden skewers, alternating the ingredients.

4. Brush the shrimp and vegetable skewers with the prepared marinade.

5. Grill the skewers for 3-4 minutes on each side, or until shrimp are pink and vegetables are tender.

6. Serve the grilled shrimp and vegetable skewers hot, garnished with fresh herbs if desired.

Nutritional Values (Approximate, per serving):

Calories: 200-250 kcal | Protein: 20-25 grams | Fat: 8-10 grams | Saturated Fat: 1-2 grams | Carbohydrates: 10-15 grams | Dietary Fiber: 4-6 grams | Sugars: 5-7 grams

Chicken and Vegetable Curry:

Prep Time: 20 minutes   **Cook Time:** 30 minutes   **Servings:** 4

Ingredients:

- 1 lb (450g) boneless, skinless chicken breasts, cut into bite-sized pieces
- 2 tablespoons olive oil
- 1 onion, diced
- 2 cloves garlic, minced
- 1 tablespoon ginger, minced
- 2 tablespoons curry powder
- 1 teaspoon ground cumin
- 1 teaspoon ground turmeric
- 1 can (14 oz) coconut milk
- 1 cup chicken broth
- 2 carrots, sliced
- 1 bell pepper, diced
- 1 zucchini, diced
- Salt and pepper, to taste
- Cooked rice, for serving
- Fresh cilantro, chopped, for garnish

Instructions:

1. Heat olive oil in a large skillet or pot over medium heat.

2. Add diced onion to the skillet and cook until softened, about 5 minutes.

3. Stir in minced garlic and minced ginger, and cook for another 1 minute until fragrant.

4. Add curry powder, ground cumin, and ground turmeric to the skillet. Cook, stirring constantly, for 1-2 minutes until spices are fragrant.

5. Add chicken pieces to the skillet and cook until browned on all sides.

6. Pour in coconut milk and chicken broth. Bring to a simmer and cook for 10 minutes.

7. Add sliced carrots, diced bell pepper, and diced zucchini to the skillet. Simmer for another 10-15 minutes, or until vegetables are tender and chicken is cooked through.

8. Season with salt and pepper to taste.

9. Serve the chicken and vegetable curry hot over cooked rice.

10. Garnish with chopped fresh cilantro before serving.

Nutritional Values (Approximate, per serving):

Calories: 300-350 kcal | Protein: 25-30 grams | Fat: 15-20 grams | Saturated Fat: 8-10 grams | Carbohydrates: 15-20 grams | Dietary Fiber: 4-6 grams | Sugars: 5-7 grams

Turkey Chili:

Prep Time: 15 minutes   **Cook Time:** 30 minutes   **Servings:** 4

Ingredients:

- 1 lb (450g) ground turkey
- 1 tablespoon olive oil
- 1 onion, diced
- 2 cloves garlic, minced
- 1 bell pepper, diced
- 1 can (14 oz) diced tomatoes
- 1 can (14 oz) kidney beans, drained and rinsed
- 1 cup corn kernels
- 2 tablespoons chili powder
- 1 teaspoon ground cumin
- 1 teaspoon paprika
- Salt and pepper, to taste
- Optional toppings: shredded cheese, diced avocado, sour cream, chopped cilantro

Instructions:

1. Heat olive oil in a large pot over medium heat.
2. Add diced onion to the pot and cook until softened, about 5 minutes.
3. Stir in minced garlic and cook for another 1 minute until fragrant.
4. Add ground turkey to the pot and cook, breaking it apart with a spoon, until browned.
5. Stir in diced bell pepper, diced tomatoes, kidney beans, corn kernels, chili powder, ground cumin, paprika, salt, and pepper.

6. Bring the chili to a simmer, then reduce heat to low and cook for 20-25 minutes, stirring occasionally.

7. Taste and adjust seasoning if necessary.

8. Serve the turkey chili hot, garnished with your choice of toppings.

Nutritional Values (Approximate, per serving):

Calories: 300-350 kcal | Protein: 25-30 grams | Fat: 10-12 grams | Saturated Fat: 2-3 grams | Carbohydrates: 25-30 grams | Dietary Fiber: 6-8 grams | Sugars: 5-7 grams

Steak Salad:

Prep Time: 15 minutes   **Cook Time:** 10 minutes   **Servings:** 4

Ingredients:

- 1 lb (450g) steak (such as sirloin or flank), grilled and sliced
- 6 cups mixed salad greens (such as spinach, arugula, and romaine)
- 1 bell pepper, sliced
- 1 cucumber, sliced
- 1 cup cherry tomatoes, halved
- 1/4 cup red onion, thinly sliced
- 1/4 cup crumbled feta cheese
- Balsamic vinaigrette dressing, for serving

Instructions:

1. Grill the steak according to your preference (medium-rare, medium, or well-done). Let it rest for a few minutes, then slice thinly against the grain.

2. In a large bowl, combine mixed salad greens, sliced bell pepper, sliced cucumber, halved cherry tomatoes, and thinly sliced red onion.

3. Arrange sliced steak on top of the salad.

4. Sprinkle crumbled feta cheese over the salad.

5. Drizzle with balsamic vinaigrette dressing just before serving.

6. Toss gently to coat everything evenly.

7. Serve the steak salad immediately as a satisfying and nutritious meal.

Nutritional Values (Approximate, per serving):

Calories: 300-350 kcal | Protein: 25-30 grams | Fat: 15-20 grams | Saturated Fat: 4-6 grams | Carbohydrates: 15-20 grams | Dietary Fiber: 4-6 grams | Sugars: 5-7 grams

CHAPTER SEVEN:

SNACKS AND DESSERTS

Banana Friands (Mini Almond Cakes):

Prep Time: 15 minutes   **Cook Time**: 15 minutes   **Servings**: 12

Ingredients:

- 4 large egg whites
- 1/2 cup (125g) unsalted butter, melted
- 1 cup (100g) almond flour
- 1/2 cup (60g) all-purpose flour
- 3/4 cup (150g) granulated sugar
- 1 ripe banana, mashed
- 1 teaspoon vanilla extract
- Confectioners' sugar, for dusting

Instructions:

1. Preheat your oven to 350°F (175°C). Grease a 12-cup mini muffin tin or friand pan.

2. In a large mixing bowl, whisk together the egg whites, melted butter, almond flour, all-purpose flour, and granulated sugar until well combined.

3. Gently fold in the mashed banana and vanilla extract until evenly incorporated.

4. Spoon the batter into the prepared muffin tin, filling each cup about three-quarters full.

5. Bake in the preheated oven for 12-15 minutes, or until the tops are golden and a toothpick inserted into the center comes out clean.

6. Remove from the oven and allow the banana friands to cool in the pan for 5 minutes.

7. Carefully transfer the friands to a wire rack to cool completely.

8. Dust with confectioners' sugar before serving.

Nutritional Values (Approximate, per serving):

Calories: 150-200 kcal | Protein: 3-5 grams | Fat: 10-12 grams | Saturated Fat: 4-6 grams | Carbohydrates: 15-20 grams | Dietary Fiber: 1-2 grams | Sugars: 10-12 grams

Berry Friands (Mini Almond Cakes):

Prep Time: 15 minutes   **Cook Time:** 15 minutes   **Servings:** 12

Ingredients:

- 4 large egg whites

- 1/2 cup (125g) unsalted butter, melted

- 1 cup (100g) almond flour

- 1/2 cup (60g) all-purpose flour

- 3/4 cup (150g) granulated sugar

- 1 cup mixed berries (such as blueberries, raspberries, and blackberries)

- 1 teaspoon vanilla extract

- Confectioners' sugar, for dusting

Instructions:

1. Preheat your oven to 350°F (175°C). Grease a 12-cup mini muffin tin or friand pan.

2. In a large mixing bowl, whisk together the egg whites, melted butter, almond flour, all-purpose flour, and granulated sugar until well combined.

3. Gently fold in the mixed berries and vanilla extract until evenly incorporated.

4. Spoon the batter into the prepared muffin tin, filling each cup about three-quarters full.

5. Bake in the preheated oven for 12-15 minutes, or until the tops are golden and a toothpick inserted into the center comes out clean.

6. Remove from the oven and allow the berry friands to cool in the pan for 5 minutes.

7. Carefully transfer the friands to a wire rack to cool completely.

8. Dust with confectioners' sugar before serving.

Nutritional Values (Approximate, per serving):

Calories: 150-200 kcal | Protein: 3-5 grams | Fat: 10-12 grams | Saturated Fat: 4-6 grams | Carbohydrates: 15-20 grams | Dietary Fiber: 1-2 grams | Sugars: 10-12 grams

Banana Fritters with Fresh Pineapple:

Prep Time: 15 minutes   **Cook Time**: 15 minutes   **Servings**: 4

Ingredients:

- 2 ripe bananas, mashed

- 1/2 cup (60g) all-purpose flour

- 2 tablespoons cornstarch

- 2 tablespoons granulated sugar

- 1/2 teaspoon baking powder

- Pinch of salt

- 1/4 cup (60ml) milk

- 1 teaspoon vanilla extract

- Vegetable oil, for frying

- Fresh pineapple slices, for serving

- Confectioners' sugar, for dusting

Instructions:

1. In a mixing bowl, combine the mashed bananas, all-purpose flour, cornstarch, granulated sugar, baking powder, salt, milk, and vanilla extract. Mix until smooth.

2. Heat vegetable oil in a deep skillet or frying pan over medium heat.

3. Drop spoonfuls of the banana batter into the hot oil, making small fritters. Fry until golden brown on both sides, about 2-3 minutes per side.

4. Remove the fritters from the oil and drain on paper towels to remove excess oil.

5. Serve the banana fritters with fresh pineapple slices.

6. Dust with confectioners' sugar before serving.

Nutritional Values (Approximate, per serving):

Calories: 200-250 kcal | Protein: 2-3 grams | Fat: 8-10 grams | Saturated Fat: 1-2 grams | Carbohydrates: 30-35 grams | Dietary Fiber: 2-3 grams | Sugars: 15-20 grams

Shortbread Fingers:

Prep Time: 10 minutes   **Cook Time:** 20 minutes   **Servings:** 12

Ingredients:

- 1 cup (225g) unsalted butter, softened
- 1/2 cup (60g) confectioners' sugar
- 2 cups (250g) all-purpose flour
- 1/4 teaspoon salt
- 1 teaspoon vanilla extract
- Granulated sugar, for sprinkling (optional)

Instructions:

1. Preheat your oven to 325°F (160°C). Line a baking sheet with parchment paper.
2. In a mixing bowl, cream together the softened butter and confectioners' sugar until light and fluffy.
3. Gradually add the all-purpose flour and salt to the creamed mixture, mixing until a dough forms.
4. Stir in the vanilla extract until well combined.
5. Press the dough into the prepared baking sheet, spreading it evenly to about 1/2 inch (1.25 cm) thickness.
6. Use a sharp knife to cut the dough into fingers or squares.
7. Optionally, sprinkle granulated sugar over the top of the shortbread fingers.
8. Bake in the preheated oven for 20-25 minutes, or until the shortbread is lightly golden.
9. Remove from the oven and let the shortbread cool on the baking sheet for 5 minutes.
10. Transfer the shortbread fingers to a wire rack to cool completely before serving.

Nutritional Values (Approximate, per serving):

Calories: 200-250 kcal | Protein: 2-3 grams | Fat: 15-20 grams | Saturated Fat: 10-12 grams | Carbohydrates: 15-20 grams | Dietary Fiber: 0-1 grams | Sugars: 5-7 grams

Caramel Nut Bars:

Prep Time: 20 minutes   **Cook Time:** 20 minutes   **Servings:** 12

Ingredients:

- 1 cup (120g) all-purpose flour

- 1/2 cup (110g) unsalted butter, melted

- 1/4 cup (50g) granulated sugar

- 1/2 cup (120g) caramel sauce

- 1 cup (120g) mixed nuts (such as almonds, pecans, and walnuts), chopped

- 1/2 cup (90g) chocolate chips

- 1/4 cup (60ml) heavy cream

- Sea salt flakes, for sprinkling

Instructions:

1. Preheat your oven to 350°F (175°C). Grease a 9x9 inch (23x23 cm) baking dish or line it with parchment paper.

2. In a mixing bowl, combine the all-purpose flour, melted butter, and granulated sugar. Mix until well combined.

3. Press the mixture evenly into the bottom of the prepared baking dish to form the crust.

4. Bake in the preheated oven for 15-20 minutes, or until the crust is lightly golden.

5. Remove from the oven and let it cool slightly.

6. Spread the caramel sauce evenly over the baked crust.

7. Sprinkle the chopped mixed nuts over the caramel layer.

8. In a small saucepan, heat the chocolate chips and heavy cream over low heat until melted and smooth, stirring constantly.

9. Pour the chocolate mixture over the nuts and caramel layer, spreading it evenly.

10. Sprinkle sea salt flakes over the top.

11. Refrigerate the bars for at least 1 hour to set.

12. Once set, cut into bars and serve.

Nutritional Values (Approximate, per serving):

Calories: 250-300 kcal | Protein: 3-5 grams | Fat: 15-20 grams | Saturated Fat: 6-8 grams | Carbohydrates: 25-30 grams | Dietary Fiber: 2-3 grams | Sugars: 15-20 grams

Chocolate-Mint Bars:

Prep Time: 20 minutes   **Cook Time**: 25 minutes   **Servings**: 12

Ingredients:

- 1 cup (120g) all-purpose flour
- 1/2 cup (110g) unsalted butter, softened
- 1/4 cup (50g) granulated sugar
- 1/4 teaspoon peppermint extract
- Green food coloring (optional)
- 1 cup (180g) chocolate chips
- 1/4 cup (60ml) heavy cream
- Confectioners' sugar, for dusting

Instructions:

1. Preheat your oven to 350°F (175°C). Grease a 9x9 inch (23x23 cm) baking dish or line it with parchment paper.

2. In a mixing bowl, cream together the softened butter and granulated sugar until light and fluffy.

3. Stir in the peppermint extract and a few drops of green food coloring, if desired.

4. Gradually add the all-purpose flour to the creamed mixture, mixing until a dough forms.

5. Press the dough evenly into the bottom of the prepared baking dish to form the crust.

6. Bake in the preheated oven for 20-25 minutes, or until the crust is lightly golden. Remove from the oven and let it cool slightly.

7. In a small saucepan, heat the chocolate chips and heavy cream over low heat until melted and smooth, stirring constantly.

8. Pour the chocolate mixture over the baked crust, spreading it evenly.

9. Refrigerate the bars for at least 1 hour to set.

10. Once set, cut into bars and dust with confectioners' sugar before serving.

Nutritional Values (Approximate, per serving):

Calories: 250-300 kcal | Protein: 2-4 grams | Fat: 15-20 grams | Saturated Fat: 8-10 grams | Carbohydrates: 25-30 grams | Dietary Fiber: 1-2 grams | Sugars: 15-20 grams

Dark Chocolate–Macadamia Nut Brownies:

Prep Time: 15 minutes   **Cook Time**: 25 minutes   **Servings**: 12

Ingredients:

- 1/2 cup (115g) unsalted butter

- 4 oz (115g) dark chocolate, chopped

- 3/4 cup (150g) granulated sugar

- 2 large eggs

- 1 teaspoon vanilla extract

- 1/2 cup (60g) all-purpose flour

- 1/4 teaspoon salt

- 1/2 cup (70g) macadamia nuts, chopped

Instructions:

1. Preheat your oven to 350°F (175°C). Grease an 8x8 inch (20x20 cm) baking dish or line it with parchment paper.

2. In a microwave-safe bowl, melt the butter and chopped dark chocolate together in short bursts, stirring occasionally until smooth.

3. In a separate mixing bowl, whisk together the granulated sugar, eggs, and vanilla extract until well combined.

4. Gradually pour the melted chocolate mixture into the egg mixture, whisking continuously.

5. Fold in the all-purpose flour and salt until just combined.

6. Stir in the chopped macadamia nuts.

7. Pour the batter into the prepared baking dish and spread it evenly.

8. Bake in the preheated oven for 20-25 minutes, or until a toothpick inserted into the center comes out with moist crumbs.

9. Remove from the oven and let the brownies cool completely in the pan before cutting into squares.

Nutritional Values (Approximate, per serving):

Calories: 250-300 kcal | Protein: 3-5 grams | Fat: 15-20 grams | Saturated Fat: 7-9 grams | Carbohydrates: 25-30 grams | Dietary Fiber: 2-3 grams | Sugars: 15-20 grams

Chocolate Truffles:

Prep Time: 20 minutes   **Chill Time:** 1 hour   **Servings**: 12 truffles

Ingredients:

- 6 oz (170g) dark chocolate, chopped

- 1/4 cup (60ml) heavy cream

- 1 tablespoon unsalted butter

- 1/2 teaspoon vanilla extract

- Cocoa powder, powdered sugar, chopped nuts, or shredded coconut for coating (optional)

Instructions:

1. Place the chopped dark chocolate in a heatproof bowl.

2. In a small saucepan, heat the heavy cream and butter over medium heat until it starts to simmer.

3. Pour the hot cream mixture over the chopped chocolate and let it sit for 1-2 minutes.

4. Stir the chocolate and cream together until smooth and well combined. If needed, microwave in short bursts to melt any remaining chocolate.

5. Stir in the vanilla extract until incorporated.

6. Cover the bowl and refrigerate the chocolate mixture for about 1 hour, or until firm enough to handle.

7. Once chilled, use a spoon or small scoop to portion out the chocolate mixture and roll it into balls.

8. Roll the truffles in cocoa powder, powdered sugar, chopped nuts, or shredded coconut, if desired.

9. Place the coated truffles on a parchment-lined baking sheet and refrigerate until firm.

10. Store the chocolate truffles in an airtight container in the refrigerator until ready to serve.

Nutritional Values (Approximate, per serving):

Calories: 100-150 kcal | Protein: 1-2 grams | Fat: 7-10 grams | Saturated Fat: 4-6 grams | Carbohydrates: 8-12 grams | Dietary Fiber: 1-2 grams | Sugars: 5-7 grams

Gingerbread Men:

Prep Time: 30 minutes   **Chill Time:** 1 hour   **Cook Time:** 10 minutes
Servings: 12 gingerbread men

Ingredients:

- 3 cups (360g) all-purpose flour

- 1 teaspoon baking soda

- 2 teaspoons ground ginger

- 1 teaspoon ground cinnamon

- 1/4 teaspoon ground cloves

- 1/4 teaspoon salt

- 1/2 cup (115g) unsalted butter, softened

- 1/2 cup (100g) granulated sugar

- 1/2 cup (120ml) molasses

- 1 large egg

- 1 teaspoon vanilla extract

- Royal icing and assorted decorations (optional)

Instructions:

1. In a mixing bowl, whisk together the all-purpose flour, baking soda, ground ginger, ground cinnamon, ground cloves, and salt until well combined. Set aside.

2. In another mixing bowl, cream together the softened butter and granulated sugar until light and fluffy.

3. Beat in the molasses, egg, and vanilla extract until smooth.

4. Gradually add the dry ingredients to the wet ingredients, mixing until a dough forms.

5. Divide the dough in half, flatten each portion into a disk, wrap in plastic wrap, and refrigerate for at least 1 hour or until firm.

6. Preheat your oven to 350°F (175°C). Line baking sheets with parchment paper.

7. On a floured surface, roll out the chilled dough to about 1/4 inch (0.6 cm) thickness. Use gingerbread man cookie cutters to cut out shapes.

8. Place the gingerbread men on the prepared baking sheets, leaving space between each cookie.

9. Bake in the preheated oven for 8-10 minutes, or until the edges are set and the cookies are firm.

10. Remove from the oven and let the gingerbread men cool on the baking sheets for 5 minutes before transferring to wire racks to cool completely.

11. Once cooled, decorate the gingerbread men with royal icing and assorted decorations, if desired.

Nutritional Values (Approximate, per serving):

Calories: 200-250 kcal | Protein: 3-4 grams | Fat: 8-10 grams | Saturated Fat: 5-7 grams | Carbohydrates: 30-35 grams | Dietary Fiber: 1-2 grams | Sugars: 15-20 grams

Irish Cream Delights:

Prep Time: 20 minutes   **Chill Time:** 2 hours   **Servings**: 12 squares

Ingredients:

- 1/2 cup (115g) unsalted butter, softened
- 1 cup (120g) confectioners' sugar
- 2 tablespoons Irish cream liqueur
- 1/2 teaspoon vanilla extract
- 1 cup (120g) graham cracker crumbs
- 1/2 cup (60g) chopped nuts (such as pecans or walnuts)
- 1/2 cup (90g) semisweet chocolate chips
- Cocoa powder, for dusting (optional)

Instructions:

1. In a mixing bowl, cream together the softened butter and confectioners' sugar until light and fluffy.
2. Stir in the Irish cream liqueur and vanilla extract until well combined.
3. Gradually mix in the graham cracker crumbs, chopped nuts, and semisweet chocolate chips until evenly distributed.
4. Line an 8x8 inch (20x20 cm) baking dish with parchment paper, leaving an overhang on the sides.
5. Press the mixture firmly and evenly into the bottom of the prepared baking dish.
6. Cover and refrigerate for at least 2 hours, or until firm.
7. Once chilled, use the parchment paper overhang to lift the Irish cream delights out of the baking dish.
8. Cut into squares and dust with cocoa powder, if desired, before serving.

Nutritional Values (Approximate, per serving):

Calories: 200-250 kcal | Protein: 2-3 grams | Fat: 15-20 grams | Saturated Fat: 7-9 grams | Carbohydrates: 15-20 grams | Dietary Fiber: 1-2 grams | Sugars: 10-15 grams

Berry and Chocolate Fudge Sundaes:

Prep Time: 15 minutes   **Cook Time:** 10 minutes   **Servings:** 4

Ingredients:

- 2 cups mixed berries (such as strawberries, raspberries, and blueberries)
- 1/4 cup (50g) granulated sugar
- 1 tablespoon lemon juice
- 1/2 cup (120ml) water
- 1/2 cup (90g) semisweet chocolate chips
- 1/4 cup (60ml) heavy cream
- Vanilla ice cream
- Whipped cream (optional)
- Chocolate shavings (optional)

Instructions:

1. In a saucepan, combine the mixed berries, granulated sugar, lemon juice, and water. Bring to a simmer over medium heat.

2. Cook the berry mixture for about 5-7 minutes, or until the berries have softened and released their juices. Remove from heat and let it cool slightly.

3. In another saucepan, heat the semisweet chocolate chips and heavy cream over low heat until melted and smooth, stirring constantly.

4. To assemble the sundaes, spoon some of the warm berry mixture into serving bowls.

5. Add a scoop of vanilla ice cream on top of the berries.

6. Drizzle the warm chocolate fudge sauce over the ice cream.

7. Optionally, top with whipped cream and chocolate shavings.

8. Serve immediately and enjoy!

Nutritional Values (Approximate, per serving):

Calories: 300-350 kcal | Protein: 3-4 grams | Fat: 15-20 grams | Saturated Fat: 8-10 grams | Carbohydrates: 40-45 grams | Dietary Fiber: 4-6 grams | Sugars: 30-35 grams

Warm Lemon Tapioca Pudding:

Prep Time: 5 minutes   **Cook Time:** 20 minutes   **Servings:** 4

Ingredients:

- 1/4 cup (45g) small tapioca pearls

- 2 cups (480ml) whole milk

- 1/4 cup (50g) granulated sugar

- Pinch of salt

- Zest of 1 lemon

- 2 tablespoons fresh lemon juice

- 1 teaspoon vanilla extract

- Fresh berries, for serving (optional)

- Mint leaves, for garnish (optional)

Instructions:

1. Rinse the tapioca pearls under cold water and drain well.

2. In a saucepan, combine the rinsed tapioca pearls, whole milk, granulated sugar, salt, and lemon zest.

3. Bring the mixture to a simmer over medium heat, stirring frequently to prevent sticking.

4. Once simmering, reduce the heat to low and continue to cook for about 15-20 minutes, or until the tapioca pearls are translucent and tender, and the mixture has thickened.

5. Remove the saucepan from the heat and stir in the fresh lemon juice and vanilla extract.

6. Let the pudding cool slightly before serving.

7. Spoon the warm lemon tapioca pudding into serving bowls.

8. Optionally, top with fresh berries and garnish with mint leaves.

9. Serve immediately and enjoy!

Nutritional Values (Approximate, per serving):

Calories: 150-200 kcal | Protein: 4-5 grams | Fat: 5-7 grams | Saturated Fat: 3-4 grams | Carbohydrates: 25-30 grams | Dietary Fiber: 1-2 grams | Sugars: 15-20 grams

White Chocolate–Mint Pots:

Prep Time: 15 minutes   **Chill Time:** 2 hours   **Servings:** 4

Ingredients:

- 6 oz (170g) white chocolate, chopped
- 1 cup (240ml) heavy cream
- 1/2 teaspoon peppermint extract
- Green food coloring (optional)
- Whipped cream, for topping (optional)
- Fresh mint leaves, for garnish (optional)

Instructions:

1. Place the chopped white chocolate in a heatproof bowl.
2. In a saucepan, heat the heavy cream over medium heat until it starts to simmer.
3. Pour the hot cream over the chopped white chocolate and let it sit for 1-2 minutes.
4. Stir the chocolate and cream together until smooth and well combined. If needed, microwave in short bursts to melt any remaining chocolate.
5. Stir in the peppermint extract and a few drops of green food coloring, if desired.
6. Divide the mixture evenly among serving cups or ramekins.
7. Cover and refrigerate the pots for at least 2 hours, or until set.
8. Once set, top with whipped cream and garnish with fresh mint leaves, if desired.
9. Serve chilled and enjoy!

Nutritional Values (Approximate, per serving):

Calories: 300-350 kcal | Protein: 2-3 grams | Fat: 20-25 grams | Saturated Fat: 12-15 grams | Carbohydrates: 25-30 grams | Dietary Fiber: 0 grams | Sugars: 20-25 grams

Cappuccino and Vanilla Bean Mousse:

Prep Time: 20 minutes   **Chill Time:** 2 hours   **Servings:** 4

Ingredients:

- 1 cup (240ml) heavy cream
- 2 tablespoons instant coffee granules
- 4 oz (115g) white chocolate, chopped
- 1 vanilla bean, split and seeds scraped
- 2 tablespoons granulated sugar
- Cocoa powder, for dusting

Instructions:

1. In a small bowl, dissolve the instant coffee granules in 2 tablespoons of hot water. Set aside to cool.
2. In a saucepan, heat the heavy cream over medium heat until it starts to simmer.
3. Remove the saucepan from the heat and stir in the chopped white chocolate until melted and smooth.
4. Stir in the vanilla bean seeds, dissolved coffee mixture, and granulated sugar until well combined.
5. Let the mixture cool slightly, then transfer it to a mixing bowl.
6. Cover and refrigerate the mousse for at least 2 hours, or until set.
7. Once set, whisk the chilled mousse until light and fluffy.
8. Divide the mousse among serving cups or glasses.
9. Dust the tops with cocoa powder before serving.
10. Serve chilled and enjoy!

Nutritional Values (Approximate, per serving):

Calories: 300-350 kcal | Protein: 2-3 grams | Fat: 25-30 grams | Saturated Fat: 15-18 grams | Carbohydrates: 20-25 grams | Dietary Fiber: 1-2 grams | Sugars: 15-20 grams

Dark Chocolate Covered Strawberries:

Prep Time: 15 minutes   **Chill Time:** 30 minutes   **Servings**: 12 strawberries

Ingredients:

- 12 large strawberries, washed and dried

- 4 oz (115g) dark chocolate, chopped

- 1 teaspoon coconut oil or vegetable shortening (optional)

- Assorted toppings (chopped nuts, shredded coconut, sprinkles), for decorating (optional)

Instructions:

1. Line a baking sheet with parchment paper or wax paper.

2. In a heatproof bowl, melt the dark chocolate in the microwave or over a double boiler, stirring occasionally until smooth. If desired, stir in the coconut oil or vegetable shortening to thin out the chocolate for easier dipping.

3. Holding each strawberry by the stem, dip it into the melted chocolate, swirling to coat evenly.

4. Allow any excess chocolate to drip back into the bowl, then place the chocolate-covered strawberry onto the prepared baking sheet.

5. If using, sprinkle the tops of the strawberries with assorted toppings while the chocolate is still wet.

6. Repeat the dipping process with the remaining strawberries.

7. Once all strawberries are dipped, place the baking sheet in the refrigerator for about 30 minutes, or until the chocolate is set.

8. Once set, transfer the chocolate-covered strawberries to a serving plate or store them in an airtight container in the refrigerator until ready to serve.

Nutritional Values (Approximate, per serving):

Calories: 50-60 kcal | Protein: 1-2 grams | Fat: 3-4 grams | Saturated Fat: 2-3 grams | Carbohydrates: 5-7 grams | Dietary Fiber: 1-2 grams | Sugars: 3-4 grams

CHAPTER EIGHT:

Tracking Your Symptoms and Progress

Tracking your symptoms and progress is essential for managing IBS effectively. Here's a structured approach to help you track your symptoms and monitor your progress:

1. **Symptom Tracking:**

   - Keep a daily journal or use a symptom tracking app to record your symptoms, including abdominal pain, bloating, diarrhea, constipation, gas, and any other relevant symptoms.

   - Note the severity of each symptom on a scale of 1 to 10, with 1 being mild and 10 being severe.

   - Record the frequency of bowel movements and any triggers that may have contributed to your symptoms (e.g., certain foods, stress, menstrual cycle).

2. **Dietary Tracking:**

   - Keep a food diary to track your daily intake of food and beverages.

   - Note any foods that trigger your symptoms and avoid or limit them in your diet.

   - Experiment with the low-FODMAP diet or other dietary interventions recommended by your healthcare provider and track how they affect your symptoms.

3. **Medication and Treatment Tracking:**

   - Keep a record of any medications, supplements, or treatments prescribed by your healthcare provider.

   - Note the dosage, frequency, and any side effects experienced.

   - Track how your medications or treatments impact your symptoms over time.

4. **Lifestyle Factors:**

   - Monitor your stress levels, sleep patterns, and physical activity.

   - Identify any lifestyle factors that may worsen or improve your symptoms.

- Practice stress-reducing techniques such as meditation, yoga, deep breathing exercises, or mindfulness to help manage stress.

5. **Progress Evaluation:**

   - Regularly review your symptom and dietary journals to identify patterns and trends.

   - Look for correlations between specific foods, activities, or events and your symptoms.

   - Discuss your progress with your healthcare provider during follow-up appointments and adjust your treatment plan as needed.

6. **Communication with Healthcare Provider:**

   - Share your symptom and progress tracking records with your healthcare provider to facilitate discussions about your condition.

   - Work collaboratively with your provider to make informed decisions about your treatment plan and lifestyle modifications.

7. **Long-Term Management:**

   - Use your tracking records to identify long-term trends and patterns in your symptoms.

   - Continuously refine your management strategies based on your experiences and insights gained from tracking.

What to avoid and what is suitable

1. **High-FODMAP Foods:** FODMAPs (fermentable oligosaccharides, disaccharides, monosaccharides, and polyols) are types of carbohydrates that may trigger IBS symptoms in some individuals. High-FODMAP foods to limit or avoid include:

   - Certain fruits: apples, pears, watermelon, mango, cherries

   - Certain vegetables: onions, garlic, cauliflower, broccoli, asparagus

   - Legumes: beans, lentils, chickpeas

   - Dairy products: milk, soft cheeses, yogurt containing lactose

   - Wheat and grains: wheat-based products, barley, rye, certain breads and cereals

2. **Gas-Producing Foods:** Some foods can cause excessive gas production and bloating in individuals with IBS. Avoid or limit:

   - Carbonated beverages

   - Cruciferous vegetables: cabbage, Brussels sprouts, kale

   - Beans and lentils

   - Onions and garlic

3. **High-Fat Foods:** High-fat foods can slow down digestion and exacerbate symptoms such as bloating and diarrhea. Limit:

   - Fried foods

   - Fatty cuts of meat

   - Creamy sauces and dressings

   - Processed foods high in trans fats

4. **Spicy Foods:** Spicy foods can irritate the digestive tract and trigger symptoms in some individuals. Avoid:

   - Hot peppers

- Spicy sauces and seasonings

- Chili peppers

5. **Caffeine and Alcohol:** These substances can stimulate the digestive system and worsen symptoms like diarrhea and abdominal pain. Limit:

- Coffee

- Tea

- Carbonated beverages

- Alcoholic drinks

Foods That Are Suitable:

1. **Low-FODMAP Foods:** Opt for low-FODMAP alternatives to reduce the risk of triggering symptoms. Suitable options include:

- Berries: strawberries, blueberries, raspberries

- Citrus fruits: oranges, lemons, limes

- Leafy greens: spinach, kale, lettuce

- Bell peppers

- Carrots

- Quinoa, rice, oats (gluten-free if sensitive)

- Lactose-free dairy products or lactose-free alternatives

2. **Lean Proteins:** Choose lean sources of protein to minimize fat intake and promote easier digestion. Suitable options include:

- Skinless poultry

- Fish

- Shellfish

- Tofu and tempeh

- Eggs

3. **Low-Fat Dairy Alternatives:** If lactose intolerant, opt for lactose-free or low-lactose dairy products such as lactose-free milk, lactose-free yogurt, or aged cheeses.

4. **Healthy Fats:** Incorporate small amounts of healthy fats into your diet from sources such as:

   - Avocado

   - Nuts and seeds (in moderation)

   - Olive oil

5. **Well-Tolerated Beverages:** Stay hydrated with water and herbal teas. Peppermint tea may help alleviate symptoms of IBS.

Low-FODMAP staples for your pastry and fridge

Low-FODMAP Staples for Your Pantry:

1. **Gluten-Free Flour Blend:** Use a blend of gluten-free flours such as rice flour, oat flour, and tapioca flour for baking low-FODMAP pastries.

2. **Baking Powder and Baking Soda:** Essential leavening agents for baking without triggering IBS symptoms.

3. **Rolled Oats:** Gluten-free rolled oats can be used in baking and breakfast recipes.

4. **Cornmeal:** Use cornmeal for making cornbread or coating baked goods.

5. **Nut and Seed Butters:** Opt for almond butter, peanut butter (without added high-FODMAP ingredients), or sunflower seed butter.

6. **Pure Maple Syrup or Rice Malt Syrup:** Natural sweeteners suitable for a low-FODMAP diet.

7. **Dark Chocolate Chips or Cocoa Powder:** Use in moderation for adding chocolate flavor to baked goods.

8. **Herbs and Spices:** Stock up on low-FODMAP herbs and spices such as cinnamon, ginger, turmeric, and vanilla extract for flavoring.

9. **Coconut Oil:** Use coconut oil as a dairy-free alternative in baking and cooking.

10. **Canned Coconut Milk:** A dairy-free alternative for creamy sauces and desserts.

Low-FODMAP Staples for Your Fridge:

1. **Eggs:** Versatile and low-FODMAP protein source for baking and cooking.

2. **Lactose-Free Milk or Plant-Based Milks:** Choose lactose-free cow's milk or plant-based alternatives such as almond milk, rice milk, or lactose-free coconut milk.

3. **Hard Cheeses:** Opt for aged hard cheeses like cheddar, Swiss, or Parmesan, which are lower in lactose.

4. **Plain Yogurt or Lactose-Free Yogurt:** Choose plain lactose-free yogurt or yogurt made from lactose-free milk.

5. **Tofu:** A versatile source of protein for savory and sweet recipes.

6. **Fresh Meat and Poultry:** Choose lean cuts of fresh meat and poultry without added marinades or sauces.

7. **Fish and Seafood:** Fresh fish and seafood are naturally low in FODMAPs and can be enjoyed in various dishes.

8. **Low-FODMAP Vegetables:** Stock up on low-FODMAP vegetables such as spinach, kale, carrots, zucchini, bell peppers, and tomatoes.

9. **Fresh Fruit:** Enjoy low-FODMAP fruits such as berries (strawberries, blueberries, raspberries), grapes, oranges, and bananas in moderation.

10. **Butter or Ghee (Lactose-Free):** Use lactose-free butter or ghee as a cooking fat.

Grains and Cereals:

1. Rice (white, brown, basmati)

2. Quinoa

3. Oats (gluten-free certified)

4. Corn (cornmeal, corn flour)

5. Buckwheat

6. Millet

Gluten-Free Flours:

7. Rice flour

8. Tapioca flour/starch

9. Potato flour/starch

10. Sorghum flour

11. Coconut flour

12. Almond flour

Breads and Wraps:

13. Gluten-free bread (check labels for high-FODMAP ingredients)

14. Corn tortillas

15. Rice cakes

16. Gluten-free wraps (made with low-FODMAP ingredients)

Pastas and Noodles:

17. Gluten-free pasta (made from rice, quinoa, corn, or chickpeas)

18. Rice noodles

Cereals and Breakfast Foods:

19. Gluten-free oats (certified gluten-free)

20. Cornflakes (without high-FODMAP additives)

21. Rice-based cereals (check labels for high-FODMAP ingredients)

22. Gluten-free granola (made with low-FODMAP ingredients)

Flavorings and Condiments:

23. Pure spices and herbs (avoid onion and garlic powder)

24. Gluten-free soy sauce (tamari)

25. Dijon mustard

26. Mayonnaise (check labels for high-FODMAP ingredients)

27. Olive oil

28. Vinegars (balsamic vinegar in small amounts)

29. Hot sauce (without high-FODMAP ingredients)

Snacks and Treats:

30. Plain potato chips

31. Popcorn (plain, air-popped)

32. Rice crackers

33. Gluten-free pretzels

34. Rice cakes with low-FODMAP toppings (e.g., peanut butter, sliced cucumber)

Dairy Alternatives:

35. Lactose-free milk (cow's milk or plant-based alternatives)

36. Lactose-free yogurt (plain or flavored)

37. Hard cheeses (cheddar, Swiss, Parmesan)

38. Dairy-free cheese alternatives (check labels for high-FODMAP ingredients)

Proteins:

39. Fresh meat (beef, chicken, turkey, pork)

40. Fresh fish and seafood

41. Tofu

42. Tempeh

Fruits:

43. Berries (strawberries, blueberries, raspberries)

44. Oranges

45. Bananas

46. Grapes

47. Kiwi

48. Pineapple (in moderation)

49. Cantaloupe

Vegetables:

50. Leafy greens (spinach, kale, lettuce)

51. Bell peppers

52. Carrots

53. Zucchini

54. Cucumber

55. Tomatoes (in moderation)

CHAPTER NINE:

Living Well with IBS

1. **Follow a Low-FODMAP Diet:** Work with a healthcare provider or dietitian to identify trigger foods and follow a low-FODMAP diet. This involves eliminating high-FODMAP foods and gradually reintroducing them to determine tolerance levels.

2. **Eat Regularly and Mindfully:** Stick to regular meal times and avoid skipping meals, as irregular eating patterns can exacerbate symptoms. Practice mindful eating by chewing food slowly, paying attention to hunger and fullness cues, and avoiding overeating.

3. **Stay Hydrated:** Drink plenty of water throughout the day to prevent dehydration and promote healthy digestion. Limit caffeinated and alcoholic beverages, as they can worsen symptoms in some individuals.

4. **Manage Stress:** Explore stress-reducing techniques such as deep breathing exercises, meditation, yoga, tai chi, or progressive muscle relaxation to help alleviate symptoms of stress and anxiety, which can trigger IBS flare-ups.

5. **Get Regular Exercise:** Engage in regular physical activity such as walking, swimming, cycling, or yoga to promote bowel regularity, reduce stress, and improve overall well-being. Aim for at least 30 minutes of moderate-intensity exercise most days of the week.

6. **Prioritize Sleep:** Establish a regular sleep schedule and aim for 7-9 hours of quality sleep each night. Practice good sleep hygiene by creating a relaxing bedtime routine, limiting screen time before bed, and creating a comfortable sleep environment.

7. **Keep a Symptom Diary:** Track your symptoms, dietary intake, stress levels, and lifestyle factors in a journal or using a symptom-tracking app. This can help you identify triggers, patterns, and trends in your symptoms, allowing for better management and treatment.

8. **Seek Support:** Connect with others who have IBS through support groups, online forums, or social media platforms to share experiences, tips, and coping strategies. Consider joining a local or virtual support group facilitated by healthcare professionals.

9. **Communicate with Healthcare Providers:** Maintain open communication with your healthcare team, including your primary care provider, gastroenterologist, and dietitian. Discuss any changes in symptoms, treatment effectiveness, or concerns you may have to receive appropriate guidance and support.

10. **Explore Treatment Options:** Work with your healthcare provider to explore various treatment options tailored to your needs, including medications, dietary supplements, probiotics, and psychological therapies such as cognitive-behavioral therapy (CBT) or gut-directed hypnotherapy.

11. **Practice Self-Care:** Incorporate self-care activities into your daily routine to nurture your physical, emotional, and mental well-being. This may include hobbies, relaxation techniques, spending time outdoors, or engaging in activities that bring you joy and fulfillment.

Future Directions and Research

1. **Microbiome Research:** Further investigation into the gut microbiome and its role in IBS holds great promise. Advances in sequencing technologies and computational analysis techniques are allowing researchers to characterize the microbiome with greater precision. Future studies may uncover specific microbial signatures associated with IBS subtypes, paving the way for personalized treatment approaches targeting the microbiota.

2. **Dietary Interventions:** While the low-FODMAP diet has shown efficacy in managing IBS symptoms for many individuals, ongoing research is needed to optimize dietary interventions. This includes exploring the long-term effects of dietary modifications, identifying additional dietary triggers beyond FODMAPs, and developing more sustainable dietary strategies that prioritize nutritional adequacy and gut health.

3. **Precision Medicine:** With advances in genetics and molecular profiling, the concept of precision medicine is gaining traction in IBS research. By integrating genetic, microbial, immune, and clinical data, researchers aim to identify biomarkers and predictive models that can inform personalized treatment decisions and improve treatment outcomes.

4. **Psychological Therapies:** Psychological factors such as stress, anxiety, and mood disorders play a significant role in IBS symptomatology. Future research may focus on developing and refining psychological interventions, such as cognitive-behavioral therapy (CBT), mindfulness-based interventions, and gut-directed hypnotherapy, to better address the psychosocial aspects of IBS and improve overall patient well-being.

5. **Neurobiological Mechanisms:** Advances in neuroimaging techniques and neurobiological research are shedding light on the complex interplay between the brain and the gut in IBS. Investigating alterations in gut-brain signaling pathways, central pain processing, and neuroimmune interactions may uncover novel therapeutic targets for symptom management.

6. **Drug Development:** Despite the growing understanding of IBS pathophysiology, there remains a significant unmet need for effective pharmacological treatments. Continued

efforts to develop targeted therapies, including novel receptor modulators, neuromodulators, and anti-inflammatory agents, hold promise for alleviating symptoms and improving quality of life for individuals with IBS.

7. **Patient-Centered Outcomes Research:** Engaging patients as partners in research is essential for ensuring that research priorities align with patient needs and preferences. Future studies may focus on patient-reported outcomes, treatment satisfaction, and the impact of IBS on quality of life, with the goal of informing patient-centered care and improving healthcare delivery.

8. **Digital Health Technologies:** The integration of digital health technologies, such as mobile apps, wearable devices, and telemedicine platforms, presents exciting opportunities for remote monitoring, symptom tracking, and patient education in IBS management. Future research may explore the effectiveness of these tools in promoting self-management and enhancing patient-provider communication.

Emerging Therapies

Emerging therapies hold promise for improving the management of Irritable Bowel Syndrome (IBS) by targeting underlying mechanisms and addressing symptomatology more effectively. Here are some noteworthy emerging therapies and treatment modalities:

1. **Microbiota-based Therapies:** Emerging evidence suggests that dysbiosis, or imbalance in the gut microbiota, may contribute to IBS pathophysiology. Microbiota-based therapies, such as fecal microbiota transplantation (FMT), microbial restoration therapy, and targeted probiotic formulations, are being investigated as potential interventions to restore microbial balance and alleviate IBS symptoms.

2. **Prebiotics:** Prebiotics are non-digestible fibers that promote the growth of beneficial bacteria in the gut. Research suggests that certain prebiotics, such as galacto-oligosaccharides (GOS) and fructo-oligosaccharides (FOS), may have therapeutic potential in IBS by modulating the gut microbiota and improving gastrointestinal function.

3. **Immune Modulators:** Abnormal immune activation and low-grade inflammation have been implicated in the pathogenesis of IBS. Immune modulators, including anti-inflammatory agents, cytokine inhibitors, and immunomodulatory drugs, are being explored as potential therapeutic targets to mitigate immune dysregulation and reduce symptom severity in IBS.

4. **Serotonin Receptor Modulators:** Serotonin (5-HT) signaling plays a crucial role in gut motility, sensation, and visceral hypersensitivity, all of which are perturbed in IBS. Novel serotonin receptor modulators, such as 5-HT3 and 5-HT4 receptor

agonists/antagonists, are under investigation for their ability to modulate gastrointestinal function and alleviate IBS symptoms.

5. **Neuromodulation:** Neuromodulation techniques, including transcutaneous electrical nerve stimulation (TENS), sacral nerve stimulation (SNS), and spinal cord stimulation (SCS), hold promise for modulating pain perception and neuronal activity in IBS. These non-invasive or minimally invasive approaches may offer alternative treatment options for individuals with refractory IBS symptoms.

6. **Peptide Therapies:** Peptides are short chains of amino acids that can exert various physiological effects in the body. Peptide-based therapies targeting gastrointestinal peptides, such as ghrelin, motilin, and neurotensin, are being investigated for their potential to regulate gut motility, appetite, and visceral sensitivity in IBS.

7. **Psychological Therapies:** Emerging psychological therapies, including acceptance and commitment therapy (ACT), gut-directed hypnotherapy, and mindfulness-based interventions, are showing promise in addressing the psychological and emotional aspects of IBS, such as anxiety, depression, and stress, which often exacerbate symptoms.

8. **Medical Foods:** Medical foods are specially formulated products intended for the dietary management of specific medical conditions. Novel medical foods designed to address the unique nutritional needs and dietary restrictions of individuals with IBS, such as low-FODMAP formulations, are being developed and evaluated for their efficacy in symptom management.

Advancements in Understanding IBS Mechanisms

1. **Gut Microbiota Dysbiosis:** Research has elucidated the role of the gut microbiota in IBS, with evidence suggesting alterations in microbial composition and function. Advancements in metagenomic sequencing and metabolomics have provided insights into specific microbial signatures associated with IBS subtypes, paving the way for microbiota-targeted therapies.

2. **Intestinal Barrier Dysfunction:** Dysfunction of the intestinal barrier, characterized by increased permeability and mucosal inflammation, has been implicated in IBS pathogenesis. Advancements in understanding the molecular mechanisms underlying barrier dysfunction, such as alterations in tight junction proteins and mucin production, are providing potential targets for therapeutic intervention.

3. **Visceral Hypersensitivity:** Heightened visceral sensitivity, or hypersensitivity, is a hallmark feature of IBS, contributing to abdominal pain and discomfort. Advancements

in neuroimaging techniques and neurobiological research have revealed alterations in central pain processing, visceral nociception, and brain-gut interactions in individuals with IBS, providing insights into the neurobiological basis of symptoms.

4. **Immune Activation:** Low-grade immune activation and immune-mediated mechanisms have been implicated in the pathophysiology of IBS. Advancements in immunological research have identified aberrant immune responses, mucosal inflammation, and cytokine dysregulation in subsets of individuals with IBS, suggesting potential targets for immune-modulating therapies.

5. **Neurotransmitter Imbalance:** Dysregulation of neurotransmitters, particularly serotonin (5-HT), dopamine, and gamma-aminobutyric acid (GABA), has been implicated in altered gut motility, sensation, and mood regulation in IBS. Advancements in pharmacological research have led to the development of novel serotonin receptor modulators and neuromodulatory agents targeting neurotransmitter pathways.

6. **Brain-Gut Axis Dysfunction:** The bidirectional communication between the brain and the gut, known as the brain-gut axis, plays a critical role in regulating gastrointestinal function and visceral sensation. Advancements in neuroimaging studies and psychophysiological research have provided insights into the complex interactions between central nervous system (CNS) activity, emotional processing, and gut physiology in IBS.

7. **Genetic and Epigenetic Factors:** Advances in genomic and epigenomic research have identified genetic predispositions and epigenetic modifications associated with IBS susceptibility and symptom severity. Genome-wide association studies (GWAS) and epigenome-wide association studies (EWAS) have uncovered genetic variants and epigenetic changes in genes related to gut function, immune regulation, and neurotransmitter signaling.

8. **Personalized Medicine Approaches:** Integration of multi-omics data, including genomics, microbiomics, metabolomics, and clinical phenotyping, holds promise for advancing personalized medicine approaches in IBS. Advancements in computational modeling, machine learning algorithms, and bioinformatics tools are enabling the development of predictive models and treatment algorithms tailored to individual patient profiles.

30-Day Low FODMAP Meal Plan

Week 1:

Day 1:

- Breakfast: Scrambled eggs with spinach and tomatoes

- Lunch: Grilled chicken salad with lettuce, cucumber, and carrots

- Dinner: Baked salmon with roasted potatoes and green beans

Day 2:

- Breakfast: Oatmeal with almond milk, banana, and a sprinkle of cinnamon

- Lunch: Turkey and cheese wrap with lettuce and bell peppers

- Dinner: Stir-fried tofu with bok choy, bell peppers, and rice noodles

Day 3:

- Breakfast: Greek yogurt with strawberries and a handful of almonds

- Lunch: Quinoa salad with mixed greens, cherry tomatoes, and grilled zucchini

- Dinner: Grilled shrimp skewers with roasted carrots and asparagus

Day 4:

- Breakfast: Smoothie made with lactose-free yogurt, blueberries, and spinach

- Lunch: Turkey and avocado sandwich on gluten-free bread with a side of baby carrots

- Dinner: Beef stir-fry with broccoli, bell peppers, and rice

Day 5:

- Breakfast: Scrambled eggs with spinach and lactose-free cheese

- Lunch: Chicken Caesar salad with homemade dressing (made without garlic)

- Dinner: Baked chicken with mashed potatoes and steamed green beans

Week 2:

Day 6:

- Breakfast: Overnight oats made with lactose-free milk, raspberries, and a drizzle of maple syrup
- Lunch: Tuna salad with lettuce wraps and sliced cucumbers
- Dinner: Grilled pork chops with roasted sweet potatoes and sautéed kale

Day 7:

- Breakfast: Smoothie bowl topped with kiwi, strawberries, and coconut flakes
- Lunch: Quinoa and roasted vegetable salad with a lemon vinaigrette
- Dinner: Baked cod with quinoa pilaf and steamed broccoli

Day 8:

- Breakfast: Scrambled eggs with spinach and lactose-free cheese
- Lunch: Turkey and cranberry wrap with lettuce and sliced bell peppers
- Dinner: Stir-fried tofu with bell peppers, carrots, and rice

Day 9:

- Breakfast: Greek yogurt with raspberries and a handful of walnuts
- Lunch: Grilled chicken salad with mixed greens, cherry tomatoes, and cucumbers
- Dinner: Baked salmon with roasted potatoes and green beans

Day 10:

- Breakfast: Oatmeal with lactose-free milk, banana, and a sprinkle of cinnamon
- Lunch: Turkey and avocado sandwich on gluten-free bread with a side of baby carrots
- Dinner: Beef stir-fry with broccoli, bell peppers, and rice

Week 3:

Day 11:

- Breakfast: Smoothie made with lactose-free yogurt, blueberries, and spinach

- Lunch: Chicken Caesar salad with homemade dressing (made without garlic)

- Dinner: Grilled shrimp skewers with roasted carrots and asparagus

Day 12:

- Breakfast: Scrambled eggs with spinach and lactose-free cheese

- Lunch: Turkey and cheese wrap with lettuce and bell peppers

- Dinner: Baked chicken with mashed potatoes and steamed green beans

Day 13:

- Breakfast: Smoothie bowl topped with kiwi, strawberries, and coconut flakes

- Lunch: Quinoa and roasted vegetable salad with a lemon vinaigrette

- Dinner: Grilled pork chops with roasted sweet potatoes and sautéed kale

Day 14:

- Breakfast: Greek yogurt with raspberries and a handful of walnuts

- Lunch: Grilled chicken salad with mixed greens, cherry tomatoes, and cucumbers

- Dinner: Baked cod with quinoa pilaf and steamed broccoli

Day 15:

- Breakfast: Oatmeal with lactose-free milk, banana, and a sprinkle of cinnamon

- Lunch: Turkey and cranberry wrap with lettuce and sliced bell peppers

- Dinner: Stir-fried tofu with bell peppers, carrots, and rice

Week 4:

Day 16:

- Breakfast: Overnight oats made with lactose-free milk, raspberries, and a drizzle of maple syrup

- Lunch: Tuna salad with lettuce wraps and sliced cucumbers

- Dinner: Grilled salmon with roasted potatoes and green beans

Day 17:

- Breakfast: Scrambled eggs with spinach and lactose-free cheese

- Lunch: Turkey and avocado sandwich on gluten-free bread with a side of baby carrots

- Dinner: Beef stir-fry with broccoli, bell peppers, and rice

Day 18:

- Breakfast: Smoothie made with lactose-free yogurt, blueberries, and spinach

- Lunch: Chicken Caesar salad with homemade dressing (made without garlic)

- Dinner: Grilled shrimp skewers with roasted carrots and asparagus

Day 19:

- Breakfast: Greek yogurt with strawberries and a handful of almonds

- Lunch: Quinoa and roasted vegetable salad with a lemon vinaigrette

- Dinner: Baked chicken with mashed potatoes and steamed green beans

Day 20:

- Breakfast: Smoothie bowl topped with kiwi, strawberries, and coconut flakes

- Lunch: Grilled chicken salad with mixed greens, cherry tomatoes, and cucumbers

- Dinner: Baked cod with quinoa pilaf and steamed broccoli

Day 21:

- Breakfast: Oatmeal with lactose-free milk, banana, and a sprinkle of cinnamon

- Lunch: Turkey and cranberry wrap with lettuce and sliced bell peppers

- Dinner: Stir-fried tofu with bell peppers, carrots, and rice

Day 22:

- Breakfast: Scrambled eggs with spinach and lactose-free cheese

- Lunch: Quinoa salad with mixed greens, cherry tomatoes, and grilled zucchini

- Dinner: Grilled pork chops with roasted sweet potatoes and sautéed kale

Day 23:

- Breakfast: Smoothie made with lactose-free yogurt, blueberries, and spinach

- Lunch: Chicken Caesar salad with homemade dressing (made without garlic)

- Dinner: Baked salmon with roasted potatoes and green beans

Day 24:

- Breakfast: Greek yogurt with raspberries and a handful of walnuts

- Lunch: Tuna salad with lettuce wraps and sliced cucumbers

- Dinner: Beef stir-fry with broccoli, bell peppers, and rice

Day 25:

- Breakfast: Overnight oats made with lactose-free milk, raspberries, and a drizzle of maple syrup

- Lunch: Turkey and cheese wrap with lettuce and bell peppers

- Dinner: Grilled shrimp skewers with roasted carrots and asparagus

Week 5:

Day 26:

- Breakfast: Smoothie bowl topped with kiwi, strawberries, and coconut flakes

- Lunch: Quinoa and roasted vegetable salad with a lemon vinaigrette

- Dinner: Baked chicken with mashed potatoes and steamed green beans

Day 27:

- Breakfast: Oatmeal with lactose-free milk, banana, and a sprinkle of cinnamon

- Lunch: Turkey and avocado sandwich on gluten-free bread with a side of baby carrots

- Dinner: Baked cod with quinoa pilaf and steamed broccoli

Day 28:

- Breakfast: Scrambled eggs with spinach and lactose-free cheese

- Lunch: Chicken Caesar salad with homemade dressing (made without garlic)

- Dinner: Grilled pork chops with roasted sweet potatoes and sautéed kale

Day 29:

- Breakfast: Greek yogurt with strawberries and a handful of almonds

- Lunch: Grilled chicken salad with mixed greens, cherry tomatoes, and cucumbers

- Dinner: Beef stir-fry with broccoli, bell peppers, and rice

Day 30:

- Breakfast: Smoothie made with lactose-free yogurt, blueberries, and spinach

- Lunch: Quinoa salad with mixed greens, cherry tomatoes, and grilled zucchini

- Dinner: Baked salmon with roasted potatoes and green beans

Conversion Table

1 teaspoon (tsp) = 5 milliliters (mL) 1 tablespoon (tbsp) = 15 milliliters (mL) 1 fluid ounce (fl oz) = 30 milliliters (mL) 1 cup (c) = 240 milliliters (mL) 1 pint (pt) = 480 milliliters (mL) 1 quart (qt) = 960 milliliters (mL) 1 gallon (gal) = 3.8 liters (L)

1 ounce (oz) = 28.35 grams (g) 1 pound (lb) = 16 ounces (oz) = 453.59 grams (g) 1 kilogram (kg) = 2.2 pounds (lbs) = 1000 grams (g)

1 inch (in) = 2.54 centimeters (cm) 1 foot (ft) = 12 inches (in) = 30.48 centimeters (cm)

1 tablespoon (tbsp) = 3 teaspoons (tsp) 1 cup (c) = 16 tablespoons (tbsp) 1 pint (pt) = 2 cups (c) 1 quart (qt) = 2 pints (pt) 1 gallon (gal) = 4 quarts (qt)